Foreword

It gives me great pleasure to introduce this revised third edition Independent First Aid at Work Training Organisations' course ma important milestones. Firstly, with the printing of this edition, the A published 50,000 copies for its members. Second, year 2002 is th of the existence of the Association. I was one of the first elected Executive Co ttee members and have enjoyed being part of its enormous growth. I have also been proud to be appointed its first President.

This manual symbolises the networking of well over 100 companies who have joined forces to work towards the maintaining of standards in First Aid training across the country and towards the mutual support of members. It has been produced by members of the Education Committee, whose aim is to try to ensure that the contents are clear, accurate and relevant to the needs of the workplace first aider. The guidelines of HSE and the Resuscitation Councils have been closely followed.

As a first aider you will hold a privileged and responsible position. Often working alone, your immediate actions will significantly affect the recovery of an ill or injured colleague. I hope you enjoy your training and wish you well in your future service as a valued first aider in the workplace.

Muireall Lawson, RGN, OHNC

President

About this Manual

This manual is designed to accompany a structured course of learning in the practice of First Aid in the Workplace, in accordance with the Health and Safety (First Aid) Regulations 1992 and the accompanying Approved Code of Practice and Guidance. It does not profess to be exhaustive, or to be the only source of reference material which could accompany such training. However, it will serve as a good aid to revision during the course and a vital source of reference in the period following first aid qualification.

The content is based on the identified competencies for First Aid at Work qualification, formulated and approved by the Association of Independent First Aid at Work Training Organisations.

It is unrealistic to expect a student to memorise all the text in this manual for assessment purposes. As an aid, the most important theory elements (underpinning knowledge) have been highlighted with a green background.

Delegate Name Sarah Hindle

Company ______________________

Course Dates 9-12th Jan 06

Index to Sections

Appendix

First Aid at Work and the Law

There are numerous regulations and laws which have a direct association with health, safety and welfare at work and the practice of first aid. A basic knowledge and understanding of these is an important foundation for the first aider.

First aid is defined as 'the first assistance or treatment given to a casualty for any injury or sudden illness before the arrival or intervention of qualified professional aid'.

The parameters of general first aid are very wide, covering a huge potential of factors such as the age of the casualty, the nature and cause of their condition, the environment and circumstances in which they are injured and the equipment and facilities which are available for treatment.

First aid at work is one particular aspect of the wider concept of first aid. That is to say, it is the practice of first aid directly associated with the hazards, risks and circumstances of the workplace and the work which is undertaken. First aid at work is just one small part of the wider subject of health, safety and welfare at work, and in Great Britain there are literally hundreds of statutory regulations which employers must, by law, abide by.

There are three main sets of health and safety legislation which directly affect first aid in the workplace. They are:

- The Health and Safety at Work etc. Act 1974;
- The Health and Safety (First Aid) Regulations 1981, as amended 1992;
- The Reporting of Injuries, Diseases and Dangerous Occurrences Regulations 1995;
- The Control of Substances Hazardous to Health Regulations 1999.

The Health & Safety at Work etc. Act 1974

This is a law which protects people at work and the general public. Under the act everyone has a legal duty to uphold certain standards of health, safety and welfare. This includes:

- employers;
- employees;
- the self-employed;
- suppliers and importers;
- those who control premises.

Duties of Employers

Under the act, employers must ensure the health, safety and welfare of their employees, so far as is reasonably practical. This means that an employer must provide employees with:

- safe equipment and working methods;
- safe arrangements for the use, handling, storage and transportation of all articles and substances;
- safe access to and from a workplace, including passages and walkways;
- a safe working environment;
- a health and safety policy if the company has five employees or more;
- protective clothing, equipment and safety devices.

Duties of Employees

All employees have a duty to take reasonable care for the health and safety of themselves and others while working. This means that as an employee you are responsible for:

- what you do - your actions;
- what you don't do - your omissions.

The Health and Safety at Work etc. Act is enforced by the Health and Safety Executive and local authorities who appoint inspectors. It is a criminal offence for an employer or self-employed person not to meet the requirements of the act and offenders may be prosecuted in the Magistrates or Crown court.

The Health and Safety (First Aid) Regulations 1981

This set of ten Regulations places a specific duty on employers and self-employed persons to ensure that they provide adequate and appropriate equipment, facilities and suitable persons for rendering first aid to employees if they are injured or become ill at work.

To help employers and self-employed people make adequate and appropriate provision, the Regulations are accompanied by an Approved Code of Practice and Guidance (ACOP). The ACOP is a lengthy document and it is unnecessary for a first aider in the workplace to be fluent with its contents. However, the first aider should have a basic knowledge and understanding.

Assessment of Need.

An employer should make an assessment of first-aid needs appropriate to the circumstances of each workplace. Based on the assessment, the employer must ensure that sufficient first-aid personnel and facilities are available whenever employees are at work.

In assessing need, employers should consider the following factors:

- workplace hazards and risks;
- the size of the organisation;
- the organisation's history of accidents;
- the nature and distribution of the workforce;
- the remoteness of the site from emergency medical services;
- the needs of travelling, remote and lone workers;
- employees working on shared or multi-occupied sites;
- annual leave and other absences of first aiders and appointed persons.

The ACOP includes a checklist to help employers assess their first aid needs.

The absolute minimum level of first-aid provision for each work site is:

- a suitably stocked and properly identified first-aid box;
- a person appointed to take charge of first-aid arrangements;
- information for employees on first-aid arrangements;

Employers and self-employed persons should be entirely familiar with the Regulations and Approved Code of Practice (ISBN 0-7176-1050-0) and if unsure about any aspect of first-aid provision for the workplace, they should contact their regional Health and Safety Executive office or local authority.

The Reporting of Injuries, Diseases and Dangerous Occurrences Regulations 1995

Reporting accidents and ill health at work is a legal requirement. The 'RIDDOR' Regulations 1995 place a legal responsibility on employers and self-employed people to make a report to their enforcing authority when certain injuries, diseases or dangerous occurrences have happened at work. The regulations state the means and time frame by which the event should be reported.

Events which must be reported include:

- Death or major injury.

  If there is an accident connected with work and an employee or a self-employed person working on the premises is killed or suffers major injury (including as a result of physical violence) or a member of the public is killed or taken to hospital

- Over three day injury.

  If there is an accident connected with work (including an act of physical violence) and an employee or self-employed person working on the premises suffers an injury which is not major but results in an injured person being away from work or unable to do their normal work for more than three days (including non-work days)

- Disease.

  If a doctor notifies an employer that an employee suffers from a reportable work-related disease

- Dangerous occurrence.

  If something happens which does not result in a reportable injury, but which clearly could have done, then it may be a dangerous occurrence

Employers should keep a full record of any injury, disease or dangerous occurrence. This must include the date and method of reporting, the date, time and place of the event, personal details of those involved and a brief description of the nature of the event or disease.

Employers and self-employed persons should be entirely familiar with RIDDOR Regulations (ISBN 0-7176-1012-8) and if unsure about any aspect of accident/occurrence reporting for the workplace, they should contact their regional Health and Safety Executive office or local authority.

The Control of Substances Hazardous to Health Regulations 1999

Under these regulations the employer has a legal duty to assess the risk of infection for employees and others affected by their work. Employees must have suitable training and take suitable precautions to protect their health, as necessary.

With regard to first aid, this book gives advice on good hygiene practice and avoiding contamination with such hazards as blood-borne viruses (see section 10.6). If the initial risk assessment indicates a need, immunisation should be offered free of charge to first aiders. It is not normally necessary to be immunised.

Employers are required to have a code of practice for dealing with spillages and other forms of contamination, of which first aiders should make themselves aware. It should be noted that a puncture wound from a needle known to contain blood contaminated with a blood-borne virus should be reported as a dangerous occurrence.

Employers should facilitate people with a blood-borne virus to work normally, unless they become unfit to do their job. There is no onus on the individual to report that they suffer from a blood-borne virus and they have a right to confidentiality.

Criminal and Civil Law

Any person who practises first-aid on a voluntary or professional basis must have an understanding of criminal and civil laws which may have a bearing on their actions.

1. Sexual Assault

It is an essential element of all first aid treatments to respect the dignity of the casualty and try to incorporate a high degree of confidentiality and respect in any care that is given. In the main, first aid includes an element of contact with a casualty, and in some cases this may mean touching the casualty in sensitive or private areas of their body, for example the groin or breast area. If the casualty has to be touched in such an area, the first aider is advised to have a witness present who can vouch for the fact that the level of contact was the minimum necessary for good treatment of the casualty and that it was carried out in a clinical manner, conducive with first-aid practice.

In some cases, it may be practicable to ensure that the first aider is the same sex as the casualty.

2. Common Assault

In some cases, just the physical act of touching an injured person without their consent or permission can present a potential problem which technically can be interpreted as common assault. It is generally accepted in first aid that, in the absence of any objection, the casualty gives their consent for treatment. In some cases the casualty may be unconscious and unable to raise any objection, therefore it is perfectly acceptable for the first aider in the workplace to administer necessary treatment.

If a conscious casualty should refuse treatment by a first aider in the workplace, the first aider should immediately refer the situation to their supervisor or manager and, if possible, get another first aider or bystander to vouch for the fact that treatment was refused. Details relating to the accident, any injuries sustained and the fact that treatment was refused must still be recorded in the accident book (see section 23).

3. Trespass/Theft

In some instances, particularly when dealing with an unconscious casualty, it may be necessary to remove any bulky or potentially harmful objects from a casualty's person, e.g. from a pocket. If this is the case, and to remove any question of wrong doing, it is advised that, if possible, the first aider have their actions witnessed by another first aider or bystander. Any personal effects which are removed from a casualty's possession, including spectacles and dentures, should be placed inside a suitable container, e.g. an envelope, and passed on to the emergency services when they arrive. If appropriate and time permits, it is also a good idea to write an inventory of contents and label the container with the casualty's personal details.

4. Negligence

Negligence exists where:

- there is a duty of care;
- there is a breach of that duty;
- harm results.

As the appointed first aider at work, you have a duty of care to employees or to members of the public affected by your employer's work and who are involved in an accident.

The most obvious breach of duty of care is failing to attend an accident. It is therefore imperative that if there is a call for a first aider, then you must attend.

There is another possible breach of duty of care, and this may occur if you do not maintain your standard of first aid at the required level. For example, moving a casualty unnecessarily before ascertaining the presence of a back injury could be a breach of duty of care.

Finally, of course, harm must result. Since the aim of first aid is to be of benefit to the casualty, it follows that if you do not attend or you do the wrong thing, harm may result.

Introduction to First Aid

Before the practice of first aid can begin, it is essential that knowledge relating to the role and responsibilities of the first aider are understood

The Responsibilities of a First Aider

There are five main responsibilities which face a first aider in the workplace:

- Assess
- Diagnose
- Treat
- Dispose
- Record

Assess

On arrival at the scene of an accident, it is essential that a quick but thorough assessment is made relating to many factors:

1. What happened?

Quickly determine the nature and circumstances of the accident.

2. Is the area safe?

Assess the area for any danger which may be present. If the situation dictates that there is further danger to the first aider or casualty then there are three courses of action to consider:

a. Stay away.

If the danger is extreme or beyond the first aider's ability to cope, the best course of action is to keep well clear and leave the situation to qualified professional help. Do not become a casualty yourself!

b. Move the danger.

In some situations it may be possible to remove or isolate the danger at the scene of an accident, e.g. to turn off an electricity supply or to move an object which presents a falling or trip hazard. This method of dealing with danger is often the best as it does not involve moving the casualty from the scene, which could potentially make the casualty's condition worse.

c. Move the casualty.

In some situations it may be very difficult or impossible to remove or neutralise danger at the scene of an accident. If this is so, it may be necessary to remove the casualty from the source of danger. When this course of action is taken, try to minimise the risk of causing any further injury to the casualty by moving them carefully and, where possible, utilising the help of bystanders.

3. How many casualties are there?

The accident may have given rise to several different casualties. If the history of the accident indicates that multiple casualties are possible, a quick sweep around the area should be undertaken to ensure all injured persons are accounted for. It may be possible to ask bystanders or casualties how many people were present at the accident area.

4. Do I need help?

In some cases, the nature and magnitude of the incident may dictate that immediate help in the local vicinity is required. In many cases there may be bystanders who can help but in circumstances where the first aider is alone it may be necessary to shout for help. When the first aider is making their initial assessment at the scene of an accident it is very important that they remain calm and collected and do not add to any panic or confusion which may already be evident. It is often a good idea to introduce yourself as a first aider as you arrive on the scene as this can help instil confidence and co-operation in others.

Diagnose

Before any definitive treatment can be given to a

casualty it is essential to evaluate their condition. This is called a diagnosis. There are three elements to consider when forming a diagnosis:

1. History

This means how and when the accident or illness occurred. In some cases the cause and nature of the accident may be obvious but in some cases it may not. Bystanders at the scene of an accident may be able to tell you what happened or may even be able to tell you of any underlying medical condition from which the casualty is suffering. Clues may be evident which point toward a particular cause of injury or illness. Information regarding the cause and circumstances of the accident can be of considerable help in finding and diagnosing a casualty's condition. Think back to when you have been examined by a G.P. or casualty department doctor and the odds are that the first question they asked you was "How did you do this?"

Things to look for include:

- History of impact or violence to the casualty.
- Evidence of electrocution or contact with a chemical substance.
- Machinery or tools which the casualty may have been using.
- Evidence of smoke or other harmful substances.
- The history of an accident can give a very good indication as to the nature and severity of injuries which a casualty has sustained.

2. Signs

All injuries and illnesses have particular pointers or features which may help with the diagnosis. Signs of injury or illness are the features discovered by applying four of your five senses when examining the casualty.

a. Look:

At the site of injury for swelling, deformity, unusual movement, bruising, foreign bodies, bleeding. At the casualty in general for anxiety or stress, painful expression, sweating, difficult or laboured breathing, abnormal skin colour, incontinence, injection/sting/bite marks, vomiting, any other signs of injury.

b. Listen:

For any unusual breathing sounds, to the legibility and clarity of the casualty's speech, to any statements made by the casualty or bystanders.

c. Feel:

For deformity of the bone structure, dampness in the groin region, skin temperature, tenderness, swelling.

d. Smell:

The casualty's breath for acetone (sweet smell) or alcohol.

3. Symptoms

These are the sensations and feelings which the casualty has or may be able to describe to you. For example, the exact location of pain, weakness or paralysis, temperature and dizziness. You may need to ask questions to establish the presence or absence of some symptoms.

Useful questions for questioning a conscious casualty:

Q - What happened?

Is the response clear? Confused? Incomprehensible?

Q - What is your name?

Is the response clear? Confused? Incomprehensible?

Q - Exactly where is the pain?

Is the casualty capable of moving by themselves to indicate the area?

Q - Are you taking any medication or being seen by a doctor for any medical condition?

Q - Have you ever had this problem before? (In cases of suspected medical conditions.)

If yes, when? How often? Is it worse than last time?

Q - Are you allergic to anything?

Q - Is there anyone else I should inform about your condition? e.g. relative, work.

Remember :

HISTORY + SIGNS + SYMPTOMS = DIAGNOSIS

Treat

The main aims of first-aid treatment for any injury or medical condition are to :

- Save life.
- Prevent the condition from becoming worse.

P - prevent P - promote

P - preserve

1. **To Save Life**

   Knowing that your skills could save another person's life is a great incentive for learning. Even in a very hazardous working environment, situations where a person's life is at risk are not commonplace; indeed, the vast majority of first aiders may never deal with anything more serious than a broken ankle or a small cut. This statistic, however, does not mean that a first aider should ignore the possibility (no matter how remote) that they may at some time have to provide life saving treatments. Being prepared for the worst is very important.

2. **To Prevent the Condition Becoming Worse**

   When a person is injured or ill, their condition can be classified into one of three possible states. It could be deteriorating (getting worse), stabilised (remaining constant) or improving (getting better). If the first aider can stop, or at least slow down, the speed of deterioration in the casualty's condition, it could give the casualty a few more precious minutes which could mean the difference between life or death. This idea is best demonstrated by means of a graph.

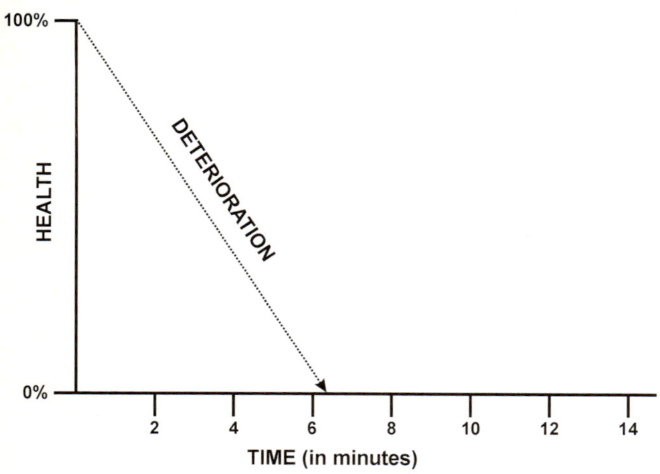

GRAPH 1 - Without Treatment

The first graph represents the conditional status of a casualty who is bleeding from a major open wound. It shows that without treatment the casualty will continue to deteriorate and eventually reach 0% health (or death) in six minutes.

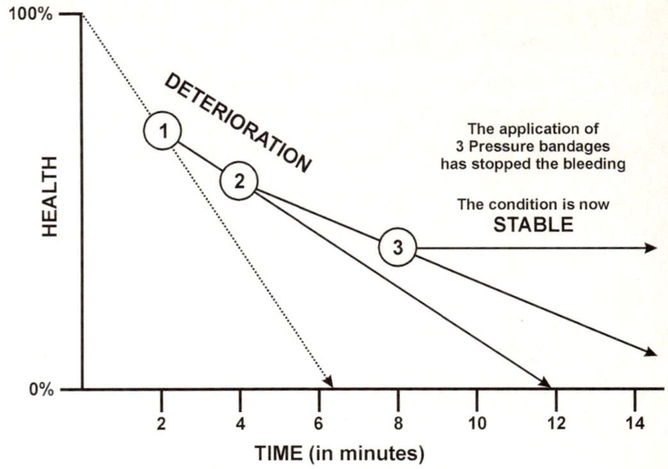

GRAPH 2 - With Treatment

The second graph shows that at 2 minutes the casualty received some treatment for the bleeding (in this case the application of a pressure bandage over the wound) and this has an immediate effect. Although the casualty is still deteriorating, the speed of deterioration is less. Good observation of the casualty shows that by 4 minutes blood has seeped through the initial dressing so a second pressure dressing has been applied on top of the first. This extra pressure has slowed the bleeding down even further. Once again, good observation shows that by 8 minutes blood has seeped through the second dressing so a third pressure dressing is applied directly over the top of the second. Although still very serious, the casualty's condition is now stable. Overall conclusion - without treatment the casualty will die within 6 minutes, with treatment the casualty will still be alive when the emergency medical aid arrives.

Good first aid can, in some cases, actually result in a slight improvement of the casualty's condition although full recovery may take weeks or even years, depending on the nature and severity of the problem. There are some casualties for whom first aid is of little benefit, simply because their injury or condition is so severe. Even so, a first aider should always do their best regardless of how pointless the task appears. There have been many cases where even qualified doctors have given a patient little or no hope of survival only to be proved wrong!

In some cases, the only treatment a first aider in the workplace can give is simple advice to the casualty. Take, for example, a casualty who complains of toothache. There is no specific treatment for this condition and in most circumstances all the first aider can do is offer advice to the casualty to the effect of "If the pain persists or gets worse, go see your dentist". Although no physical treatment has taken place, the fact that a person reported to the first aider with a problem should still be recorded, alongside any advice that the first aider gave. Who knows, maybe frequent aches and pains (including headaches) are the result of an environmental problem which secretly exists in the workplace? If all details are recorded, the company health and safety manager can identify the problem and, if necessary, investigate possible causes within the work-place.

In some instances, the first aider may have to deal with more than one casualty or a single casualty with more than one injury. If this is the case it is important that treatments are prioritised, thus ensuring that the most serious injuries and conditions are treated first, and leaving minor injuries and conditions until last.

A basic but highly endorsed system of prioritisation is known as the A.B.C system.

Life threatening injuries and conditions should be prioritised in the following order:

1st **Airway.** Any condition which causes blockage or obstruction to the main breathing tubes of the respiratory system, particularly the mouth and throat (see section 3).

2nd **Breathing.** Any condition which causes stoppage or interference with the mechanism of breathing.

3rd **Circulation.** Any condition which causes stoppage or interference with the circulation of blood around the body (see section 4).

Non-life-threatening injuries and conditions should be prioritised in the following order:

1st Those likely to result in the deterioration of a casualty's condition, possibly to a life-threatening extent before the arrival of further medical aid.

2nd Those likely to result in no deterioration of a casualty's condition.

Dispose

This means the course of action to be taken after treatment by the first aider. There are many potential methods of casualty disposal which a first aider may consider:

1. Return to Work

In the majority of cases following minor injury, a casualty may return to work after treatment. If this is the case, however, the casualty should always be advised to report back to the first aider or their doctor if the condition appears to worsen. A good example of this is a small 'paper cut'. Having received treatment by the first aider, it may be that throughout the day the cut still bleeds slightly or, over the next few days, perhaps becomes infected. A good first aider should always think carefully about the potential long term development of further problems arising with the condition (this is referred to as the prognosis) and advise the casualty accordingly. As already mentioned, the advice given to the casualty should also be recorded alongside any physical treatments which were given.

2. To see their own or company doctor

Some casualties may need to see a doctor shortly after injury or sudden illness even though the condition does not constitute an emergency . A good example of this is where a casualty has sustained a small open wound which is particularly dirty and fresh water alone is not adequate to deal with the potential infection (or perhaps the casualty may need a tetanus injection). Cleaning of wounds with antiseptic solutions or creams is well beyond the normal scope of first aid in the workplace and therefore, unless specifically trained and deemed competent, a first aider should not attempt to use any medications to clean wounds. (Solutions and creams can also cause allergic reactions.) This is the responsibility of the casualty's own doctor's surgery, or if available, their company's Occupational Health department or nurse. If a visit to their own doctor is difficult at short notice, the casualty department of the local hospital should be considered, although treatment of this type of problem will take a very low priority.

3. Taken to Hospital (Non-emergency)

Although again not an emergency, a casualty's condition may often warrant further investigation and treatment from the casualty department of the local hospital. An example of this is a suspected broken hand or fingers. First-aid treatment can often be sufficient to stabilise the injury short term but the casualty will certainly need to be seen at hospital. Taken to hospital means exactly that - the casualty is escorted all the way, not just told to make their own way. Just imagine the consequences if a person with broken fingers tried to drive themselves to hospital!

4. Taken to Hospital (Emergency)

The only way that a casualty should be taken to hospital in an emergency situation is by an ambulance.

When calling for an ambulance the following information should be given in a clear, unhurried and logical sequence:

a. Confirmation of the telephone number from which the call is being made.
b. The name of the caller.
c. The exact location of the incident.
d. The nature or cause of the incident.
e. How many casualties there are and information relating to their general diagnosis.
f. What first aid treatments have already been administered.

The operator may ask other questions relating to the incident so it is important that the person making the call is familiar with the incident. When all information is passed, the operator may give an indication as to how long the ambulance may take to arrive. When finished, the operator should be the one to terminate the call.

If a bystander is used to make the call, it may be necessary for them to write down certain details to ensure that the information given is correct and the bystander should be told to report back to the first aider when the call has been made.

In all cases where an emergency ambulance has been called to the workplace, the first aider should ensure that their supervisor or line manager is informed of the occurrence at the earliest possible opportunity.

In many cases, the ambulance service may be able to give the first aider further advice regarding the treatment and disposal of the casualty.

Record

All accidents in the workplace (even those where nobody was injured) have to be recorded in the accident book (see section 23).

Test Your Knowledge

1) You are on your own and arrive at the scene of an accident involving 3 casualties:

   a) one person lying down, sobbing and obviously in severe pain
   b) one person who is sitting and is bleeding from a wound to the forearm
   c) one person with no obvious injuries who is lying face up and unconscious

   State which order you should prioritise these: a) .... b) .... c) ....

2) In order to be able to survive, a person must have:

   i A..
   ii B..
   iii C..

3) The first and most important thing you should do on arrival at the scene of an accident is to (please tick one answer):

   a) check the airway of the casualty
   b) check for dangers
   c) phone for an ambulance
   d) control severe bleeding

The Respiratory System

The breathing process is an essential element in the support of human life. It is therefore important that a first aider has a basic understanding of the respiratory process.

The human body is made up of billions of individual building blocks called cells. There are many different types of cell, different in size, different in shape, different in function, but all living cells in the body have one thing in common - they all need a constant and adequate supply of oxygen (O_2) to stay alive. Different cells have different tolerance levels to a lack of oxygen. Skin and muscle cells, for example, can last for around one hour without an oxygen supply before under-oxygenation becomes a problem. Brain cells on the other hand would generally die within eight minutes of oxygen deprivation. The air around us usually contains more than enough oxygen to support life. In fact at sea level, under normal atmospheric conditions, approximately one fifth of the air we breathe is oxygen. The body only absorbs about a quarter of this.

When body cells use oxygen (and nutrients such as proteins and fats), waste products are formed as a result of the intra-cellular chemical processes. Some waste products are in solid or liquid form and some are in gaseous form. The main waste gas produced whenever cells assimilate oxygen is called carbon dioxide (CO_2).

The function of the respiratory or breathing system is twofold. Firstly, to supply the body with the oxygen it needs from the surrounding air, and secondly (and just as important), to rid the body of excess amounts of carbon dioxide. The process of inspiration (breathing in) supplies the oxygen and the process of expiration (breathing out) expels the excess carbon dioxide.

Organs and Structures of Respiration

The main component parts of the respiratory system are as follows:

1. **The Nose and Mouth**
   The entry ports for air into the body.

2. **The Throat (Pharynx)**
   This is where the nose and mouth passages meet.

3. **The Voice Box (Larynx)**
   The hard, cartilaginous area of the upper trachea.

4. **The Windpipe (Trachea)**

5. **The Bronchi**
   Two tubes which branch off the trachea and enter the lung tissue.

6. **The Bronchioles**
   Hundreds of thousands of small tubes branching off each other and getting smaller and smaller as they get deeper into the lung tissue. Most have a diameter of between 0.5mm and 0.1 mm.

7. **The Alveoli**
   Millions of tiny air sacs which form the end of the respiratory tree. It is in the alveoli where the oxygen in the inspired air is absorbed into the blood stream and the excess carbon dioxide in the blood stream is passed into the alveoli ready for exhalation.

8. **The Pleural Space**
   This is the space or area between the outside of the lung and the inside of the chest wall. It is lined by a membrane called the pleura.

9. **The Chest Wall**
   This robust yet surprisingly flexible structure is mainly comprised of ribs (12 pairs), connective muscles (intercostals) and other soft tissue.

10. **The Diaphragm**
    This is a large sheet of muscle which forms the lower boundary of the chest cavity and the upper boundary of the abdominal cavity. It is the main muscle of respiration and breathing would be impossible without it. In its relaxed position it is a dome shape.

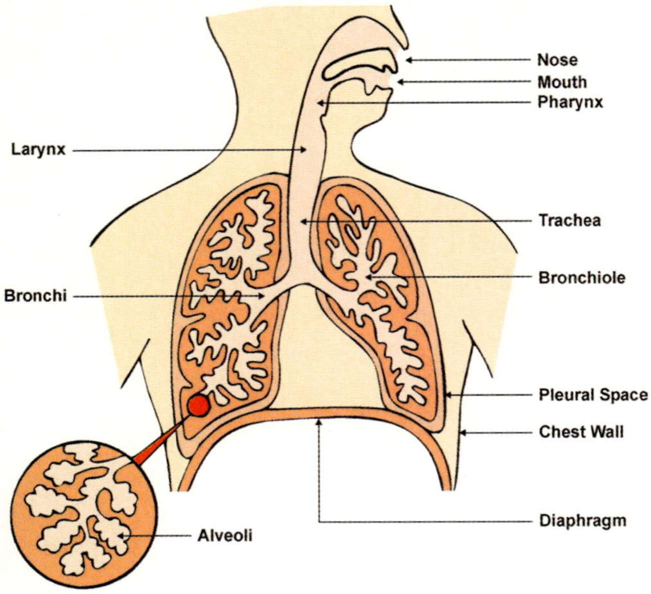

Fig.1. Organs and Structures of the Respiratory System

The Mechanism of Normal Breathing

The normal breathing cycle comprises three phases: Inspiration, Expiration and a brief Pause before the cycle repeats itself. The normal speed of breathing for a healthy adult at rest is between 14 to 18 cycles per minute. Each normal breath for an adult will inhale and exhale approximately 250ml of air.

1. Inspiration

Breathing in requires the contraction of specific muscles around and within the chest cavity.

a. The Intercostals

The intercostal muscles connect the ribs together and when they contract they change the shape of the chest cavity. The rib cage, especially the central and lower portion, is particularly flexible. The ribs are connected to the frontal aspect of the chest at the sternum (breastbone) and to the rear aspect at the spine. In their normal resting position these curved bones slope downward. When the intercostal muscles contract the ribs are lifted upward and, due to the curved shape, the sides of the chest expand outward (just like a bucket handle).

The lungs are attached to the inside of the chest wall by two layers of tissue called pleura (the space between the layers is referred to as the pleural space). The outward movement of the chest wall therefore helps the lungs to expand.

b. The Diaphragm

The diaphragm is a large sheet of muscle which forms the lower boundary of the chest cavity. In its normal relaxed position, the diaphragm adopts a curved or domed shape which roughly follows the curved line of the lower ribs. When the diaphragm contracts it changes shape by pulling down and flattening (thus pressing on the upper abdominal organs).

On inspiration, the muscular contractions of the intercostals and diaphragm enlarge the chest cavity. This causes a negative pressure (vacuum) to occur inside the chest cavity. Under normal circumstances, the only way the negative pressure can be equalised is to draw air in through the nose and mouth and into the lungs. This causes the lungs to inflate.

2. Expiration

On expiration, the relaxation of the intercostals and diaphragm reduce the size of the chest cavity. This causes a positive pressure to occur inside the chest cavity. Under normal circumstances, the only way the positive pressure can be equalised is to force air out of the lung. This causes the lung to deflate.

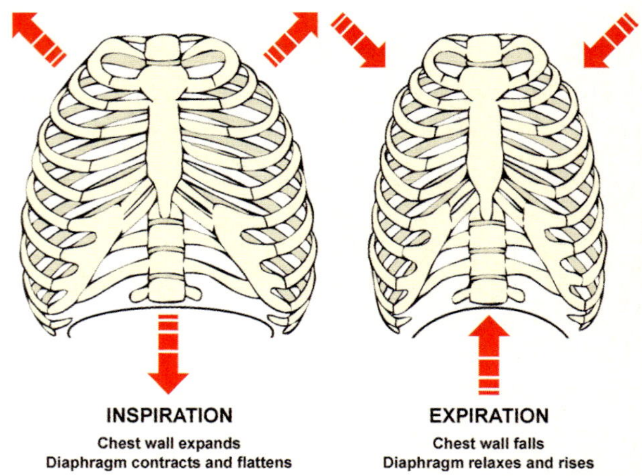

Fig.2. The Mechanism of Breathing

The breathing process would be severely hindered if:

- The chest wall is damaged or compromised.
- Movement of the chest wall is restricted.
- The airway passages are blocked.

Gaseous Exchange

The air around us which we breathe is comprised of many different gases. At normal atmospheric pressure (e.g. sea level), air is made up of approximately:

a.	**Oxygen**	-	21%
b.	**Carbon dioxide**	-	1%
c.	**Nitrogen**	-	77%
d.	**Other Gases**	-	1%

Every time we breathe, these quantities of gas are taken into the lungs. As we already know, we breathe to take in oxygen and to rid the body of excess carbon dioxide so the quantities of gas which are exhaled will be slightly different:

a.	**Oxygen**	-	17%
b.	**Carbon dioxide**	-	5%
c.	**Nitrogen**	-	77%
d.	**Other Gases**	-	1%

As you can see from the above figures, the expired air has more carbon dioxide and less oxygen but the values of the nitrogen and inert gases remain the same.

- We only use a fifth of the oxygen that we breathe in.
- We therefore exhale sufficient oxygen to give to a non-breathing person in the form of artificial ventilation (mouth-to-mouth).

The small amount of oxygen which is not exhaled (about one quarter of that inhaled) will absorb through the very thin walls of the alveoli and into the blood stream in the lungs.

At the same time as oxygen is passing from the alveoli into the blood stream, excess carbon dioxide in the blood stream is passing into the alveoli ready to be excreted on the next exhalation.

Test Your Knowledge

1) How much oxygen is in the air you breathe out (please tick one answer):

a) 10% b) 17%
c) 20% d) 27%

2) How much of the oxygen which you breathe in do you use (please tick one answer):

a) a third b) half
c) a fifth d) a quarter

3) Name three parts of the respiratory system:

a) ....

b) ....

c) ....

The Circulatory System

The circulatory system is one of the main elements of the body. Many injuries and medical conditions have a direct influence on the way the system works.

The function of the circulatory system is to carry blood around the body. Circulating blood has many important tasks to perform, such as:

- Transportation of oxygen and nutrients to all body tissues and cells.
- Transportation of waste products away from body tissues and cells (e.g. carbon dioxide).
- Transportation of chemical substances around the body (e.g. hormones).
- Assisting with the body's defence mechanism against infection.
- Assisting with the regulation of body temperature.

Organs and Structures of the Circulatory System

1. The Heart

The heart is a hollow, muscular organ which is responsible for pumping blood around the body. It is located behind the breastbone and between the two lungs.

The heart is divided into four main chambers, (2 on the left and 2 on the right). Inside the heart, a series of non-return valves separate the four chambers to ensure that blood can only flow in one direction through the heart.

De-oxygenated blood from the body tissues enters the heart in the upper right chamber from where it is pumped into the lower right chamber.

From here the blood is pumped to the lungs where the gaseous exchange process takes place in the alveoli. Oxygenated blood from the lungs is then returned to the upper left chamber of the heart from where it is pumped to the lower left chamber. From here it is pumped out of the heart on its way to the body tissues and cells. This process of blood flow through the heart is called the cardiac cycle (see fig. 3).

The cardiac cycle is a very complex system which relies on the perfect co-ordination of electrical and mechanical actions. The heart chambers must contract or pump in a particular sequence, speed and strength to ensure adequate circulation is achieved.

The normal cardiac or heart rate for a healthy adult at rest is between 60 to 80 cycles (or beats) per minute. Many injuries and medical conditions have an adverse influence on the heart beat, affecting its speed, strength and regularity.

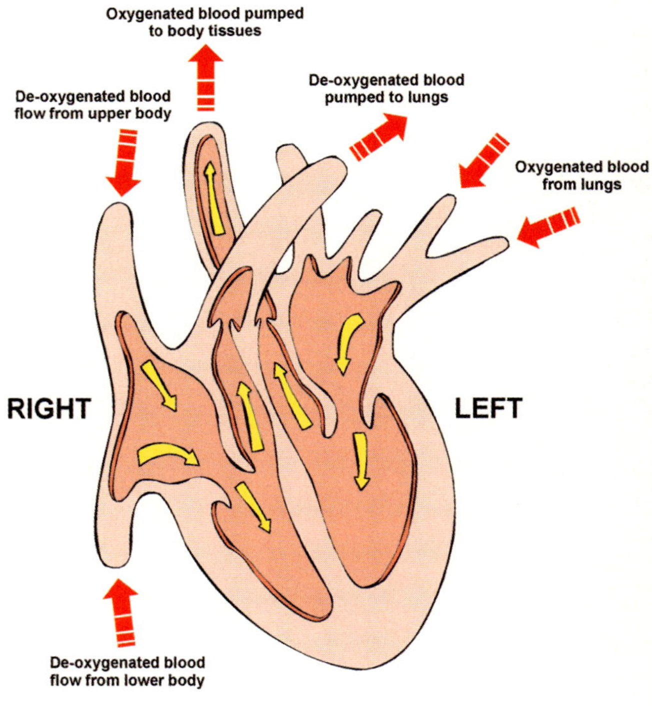

Fig.3. The Cardiac Cycle

2. Blood Vessels

Blood vessels can be found all over the body: there are millions of them. They fall into three main categories: arteries, veins and capillaries. The function of all blood vessels is to carry blood around the body.

a. Arteries

These are thick walled muscular tubes which carry blood away from the heart to all parts of the body.

The thick, muscular walls are required to withstand the pressure of the pumping blood inside. One very large artery exits from the heart (the aorta). Other smaller arteries branch off the aorta and then smaller arteries branch off these. Eventually this branching off system results in tiny arteries called arterioles spreading in a very intricate network through most of the body tissue. Some first aid procedures, such as pulses and pressure points, require pressure to be applied to main arteries in the body, therefore a first aider must be familiar with their locations:

i. The Carotid Artery

There are two carotid arteries, one either side of the upper windpipe. They carry oxygenated blood to the head and brain and therefore have extreme importance.

ii. The Brachial Artery

The brachial artery runs down the length of the upper arm bone (humerus) on the inner aspect. Its main protection is from the humerus bone and the upper arm muscles.

iii. The Radial Artery

The radial artery branches off the brachial artery at the elbow. It runs from the elbow joint to the hand. It usually lies deep inside the lower arm muscles but it does come close to the surface of the skin on the thumb side of the wrist.

iv. The Femoral Artery

The femoral artery runs from the groin region, down the upper leg to the back of the knee. In the main it is situated deep in the upper leg muscle, protected by the muscle and upper leg bone (femur). It does, however, come close to the surface of the skin in the groin area

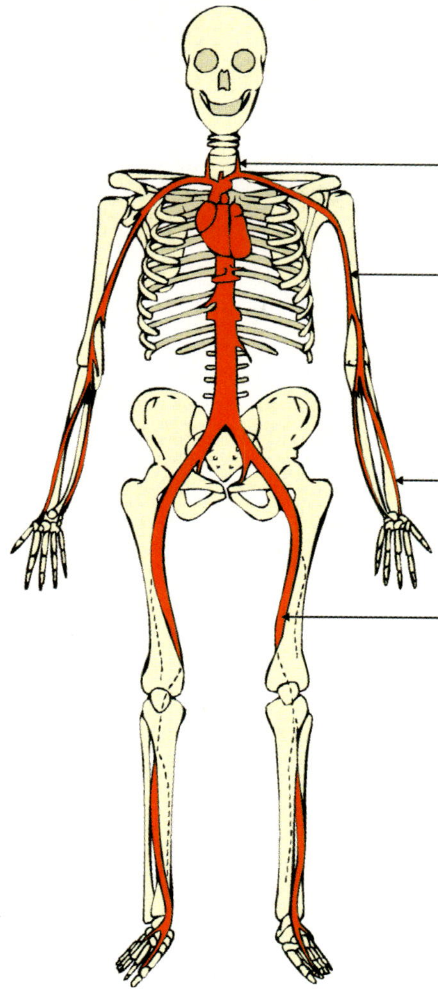

Fig.4. Main Arteries used in First Aid

The blood inside the arteries is pressurised. This pressure ensures that the blood can be forced all the way to the tiny capillaries in the extremities and vital organs. The blood pressure also ensures that blood vessels remain in their open, tube shape. If the pressure of blood should drop in the arteries, (e.g. due to blood loss) all blood vessels begin to collapse. This means that blood can no longer flow through them and oxygen supply to tissues and the organs is severely restricted.

The Pulse

Every time the heart beats, a pressure wave of blood is pumped around the body in the arteries. If firm but gentle pressure is applied to an artery, especially in an area where the artery passes over a bone close to the surface of the skin, the rhythmic expansion of the artery can be felt. This is known as the pulse and is a very accurate reflection of the speed, power and regularity of the cardiac cycle.

Although pulses can be felt in many parts of the body, first aiders usually confine themselves to four main ones which can be found on the four main arteries listed above.

i. The Carotid pulse can be found by pressing on the carotid artery in the neck. Usually at the level of the Adam's apple, between the windpipe and the adjoining neck muscle.

ii. The Brachial pulse can be found by pressing on the brachial artery in the upper arm. Usually in the middle of the artery, between the humerus bone and the upper arm muscle.

iii. The Radial pulse can be found by pressing on the radial artery on the thumb side of the wrist.

iv. The Femoral pulse can be found by pressing on the femoral artery in the front of the groin.

When feeling a pulse it is always best to use the tips of fingers rather than the thumb as the fingers are much more sensitive.

b. Veins

Veins are thin walled tubes which carry blood back to the heart from body tissues.

They begin as tiny tubes called venules which collect together to form larger tubes. Most veins in the body eventually connect into two very large veins which enter the upper right chamber of the heart.

The pressure of blood inside veins is usually very low, just enough pressure exists to keep the vein open in its normal tube shape. Unlike arteries, the pressure inside most veins is not sufficient to pump blood back to the heart so veins are equipped with tiny, non-return valves along their length to prevent back flow and ensure the blood only travels in the right direction. Whenever the muscles of the body contract, pressure is applied to the outer walls of veins. This squeezes the vein, pressurises the blood inside and forces the blood to circulate back to the heart.

c. Capillaries

These are minute tubes which connect the arteries to the veins.

Most capillaries have very thin outer walls which will allow gaseous exchange to take place.

3. Blood

Blood is made up of four main constituents, red cells, white cells, platelets and plasma. Blood is 45% solid and 55% liquid.

a. Red Blood Cells

These are tiny, circular, bi-concave discs which are responsible for carrying oxygen in the blood stream. They contain an iron pigment which gives them their deep red colour.

b. White Blood Cells

There are many different types of white cell in the blood. Generally they are responsible for fighting infections caused by viruses and bacteria.

c. Platelets

Platelets are a part of the blood's clotting mechanism. When blood comes into contact with air, many chemical reactions take place which make the blood begin to solidify. Platelets are a very important ingredient in this solidifying process. Without them it is very difficult for blood to clot.

d. Plasma

This liquid constituent makes up approximately 55% of the blood. When separated from the solid matter of cells and platelets it is a light yellow, straw colour. Approximately 95% of plasma is water.

The Regulation of Blood Pressure

The average adult has approximately ten pints (6 litres) of blood in their body. This blood is pressurised inside the blood vessels keeping them open and allowing for a constant and adequate circulation to all parts of the body. If blood is lost from inside the blood vessels, the internal pressure drops and blood vessels begin to collapse thus restricting flow to certain areas. As the blood flow to the cells reduces, so does the oxygen supply and cells begin to die.

When a drop in blood pressure occurs (perhaps due to bleeding), the body has a very clever and automatic response mechanism called auto-transfusion.

Some parts of the body (e.g. the vital organs) require a higher and much more constant supply of oxygen than others (e.g. the muscles of the arms and legs, the gut and the skin). When the brain senses that blood pressure is dropping (thus reducing blood flow to the vital organs) it immediately sends chemical and electrical signals to the main blood vessels in the arms, legs, gut and skin. These messages stimulate the blood vessels (peripheral circulation) to contract and close off. This reduces blood flow to these less important areas but increases the blood pressure and flow of blood to the vital organs in the abdomen, chest and head.

This pulling of blood away from the extremities causes a variety of signs and symptoms to occur such as pale, cold skin and a weak pulse.

If a reduction in blood pressure at the vital organs stimulates the influx of blood from the extremities, an increase in blood pressure will have the opposite effect. Some injuries and medical conditions, in particular those which involve direct damage to brain tissue, can cause the internal blood pressure to rise. In response to this, the body will bring the pressure down by sending blood to the extremities. This forcing of blood into the extremities causes a variety of signs and symptoms to occur such as warm, flushed skin (especially in the face) and a strong pulse.

The Regulation of Body Temperature

Another important function of blood is to help in the regulation of body temperature. The normal internal (core) body temperature is 37 degrees centigrade. This temperature is ideal for cells to grow, repair and carry out their normal functions. If the core body temperature should rise above 37 degrees C, blood vessels in the extremities begin to open up. This diverts large amounts of warm blood from the centre of the body to the outer surface where the excess heat can radiate off. This effect can especially be seen in the face, as it warms up and begins to turn red. When the core temperature returns to normal, so does the blood flow.

If the core body temperature falls below 37 degrees C, the opposite effect occurs. This time, blood vessels in the skin contract, thus pulling blood away from the surface and reducing the amount of heat which is radiated off.

By now you have probably realised that the body regulates blood pressure and temperature in a very similar way, by moving large volumes of blood from one place to another in an attempt to stabilise the problem. An understanding of this natural, self-preservation mechanism is essential as many first aid treatments are designed to assist the body in its natural reaction. If the treatment is in conflict with the body's natural reaction, the end result can be life threatening.

Test Your Knowledge

1) The normal pulse rate in an adult is (please tick one answer):

a) 10 times a minute
b) 10 per second
c) 14-18 times a minute
d) 60-80 times a minute

2) The carotid artery is in the ....
The radial artery is in the ....

3) Number these blood vessels according to the thickness of their walls (eg number the thickest No1 and so on):

a) Capillaries
b) Arteries
a) Veins

4) Which of the following statements is NOT true (please tick one answer):

a) 'Normal' temperature is 37 degrees centigrade
b) 'Normal' pulse for an adult at rest is between 60 and 80 beats a minute
c) A child's pulse rate is normally slower than an adults
d) 'Normal' respiration rate for an adult at rest is between 15 and 20 breaths a minute

Asphyxia

Asphyxia is a major cause of death at accidents and therefore has a great significance for the first aider.

The circumstances which lead to asphyxiation can be diverse but the effects are very much the same.

Definition

Asphyxia is the condition which occurs when the blood is unable to receive sufficient oxygen.

We already know that all cells in the body need oxygen to survive so asphyxia is a very serious condition. There are many reasons why the blood could be deprived of oxygen.

Causes of Asphyxia

The main common causes of asphyxiation are:

- Obstruction of the air passages.
- Damage or paralysis to the respiratory centre in the brain.
- Chest injuries/Chest fixation.
- Environmental conditions which limit the amount of oxygen in the environment.

1. Obstruction of the Air Passages

If inhaled air is unable to reach the alveoli in the lungs due to an obstruction, gaseous exchange will not be able to take place. Obstructions can occur in any of the air passages of the respiratory system but, in the majority of cases, the blockage will be in the area of the mouth or throat. Reasons why the air passages may become obstructed include:

- Foreign bodies, such as food, loose or broken teeth (including dentures).
- The tongue falling back in unconsciousness.
- Vomit, blood or saliva building up in the mouth of an unconscious casualty.
- Swelling of the air passages due to burns around the mouth or neck; for example, swallowing corrosive chemicals. Insect stings and allergic reactions around the mouth or neck can cause sufficient swelling to cause an obstruction.
- Compression or restriction around the neck (strangulation).
- Some object, external to the face, that prevents air from entering the nose or mouth (suffocation).

2. Damage/Paralysis to the Respiratory Centre in the Brain

A particular part of the brain (the respiratory centre) is responsible for ensuring that breathing occurs. If this part of the brain is damaged or its normal function interfered with, the rate, depth and regularity of breathing will be affected. Paralysis of the respiratory centre in the brain can be caused by:

- Electric shock
- Head injuries
- Poisons (including drugs)

3. Chest Injuries/Fixation of the Chest Wall

It was explained in section 3 how the breathing mechanism is dependent on the ability of a vacuum to build up inside the chest. If the chest wall is penetrated or loses its rigidity, the amount of air entering the lungs will reduce. Types of chest injuries include:

- Broken ribs (single or multiple).
- Penetrating injury.
- Rupture of lung tissue due to immense air pressure changes inside the chest cavity (mainly caused by blast).

If the chest wall is prevented from expanding, there will be insufficient room inside for the lungs to inflate and the amount of air inhaled will be reduced. This can occur when:

- The chest wall is compressed under a heavy object.
- The chest wall is compressed due to the pressure of a large crowd or mass gathering.

4. Lack of Oxygen in the Environment

In this case, air reaches the alveoli of the lungs, but for various reasons the oxygen it contains is unable to pass into the blood stream. A common cause of this is when poisonous gases are present in the air which is inhaled, such as carbon monoxide. Some poisonous gases are absorbed into the blood stream in the same way as oxygen, and they are transported to the tissues by the blood. Carbon monoxide has a much stronger affinity or magnetism to the blood than oxygen, so if equal amounts of carbon monoxide and oxygen were inhaled, all the carbon monoxide would be absorbed by the blood, leaving very little room for oxygen.

Recognition

A casualty who is suffering from asphyxia may show any or all of the following recognition points. As the asphyxia continues, these will become progressively worse.

- If the casualty is conscious, they may show signs of confusion or panic.
- The rate and depth of breathing will increase. This is the body's attempt to get more oxygen into the blood. In the latter stages the breathing may become very violent.
- As the breathing increases, it may become very noisy. If the air passages are obstructed, a whistling sound may be heard.
- Possible frothing at the mouth. When a casualty is gasping for air, he does not pause to swallow (the two actions cannot be carried out simultaneously). This leads to a build up of saliva in the mouth which becomes aerated as the casualty breathes rapidly and causes it to foam.
- Blueness of the face and lips. This is a condition known as cyanosis which indicates that the blood is not properly oxygenated. It appears earliest at the extremities of the body, such as the tips of the ears, the tip of the nose and the lips.
- Possible unconsciousness. If the amount of oxygen getting to the brain is reduced, it will interfere with its normal function. This will usually occur within 2 to 3 minutes of the brain being starved of oxygen. The development of the unconsciousness will be gradual but exactly how long it will take depends on the actual cause of the asphyxia. Inhaled poisonous gases can cause unconsciousness very quickly.

If the brain tissues become damaged due to a lack of oxygen, the damage could be permanent or even result in death.

Treatment

The main aim in the treatment of asphyxia, regardless of cause, is to increase the amount of oxygen getting into the blood stream.

- If the cause is due to an obstruction of the airway, try clearing it (see section 6).
- If the cause is due to a paralysis of the respiratory centre, carry out artificial ventilation of the lungs with exhaled air resuscitation (see section 8).
- If the cause is due to a chest injury - try to stabilise the injury (see section 15).
- If the cause is due to fixation or constriction of the chest wall - remove the constricting object and treat for any chest injury (see section 15).
- If the cause is due to a lack of oxygen in the environment - move the casualty to a better environment if possible.

Test Your Knowledge

1) Give four conditions that may cause asphyxia:

a) ....

b) ....

c) ....

d) ....

2) What signs denote lack of oxygen in the body?

a) ....

b) ....

c) ....

The Choking Casualty

Airway obstruction is a very common cause of asphyxia and death. It is therefore essential that it can be recognised and treated quickly.

The Conscious Choking Casualty

Lying behind the larynx is another tube which passes down through the neck. This is the oesophagus down which food and drink pass to the stomach. The upper aspect of the oesophagus opens out into the back of the throat just behind the top of the windpipe. One tube should carry only gas and the other should carry only solid and liquid but with the close proximity of the two tube openings there is a potential for error. To overcome this problem there is a small flap of cartilage and soft tissue located above the opening of the windpipe called the epiglottis. When we swallow the neck muscles contract and this moves the epiglottis over the top of the windpipe, sealing it off. This ensures that the swallowed substance can only pass down one of the two tubes - the oesophagus.

The swallowing reflex, although simple in design, requires a great deal of muscular co-ordination. If the co-ordination is not precise, it results in incorrect positioning of the epiglottis during the swallowing process. Therefore, when the swallowed substance reaches the back of the throat, the top of the windpipe will be slightly open and the substance will enter the air passage (it's gone down the wrong hole).

The passage of a solid or liquid substance into the top of the windpipe causes a massive and quite dramatic response. Firstly, the neck muscles go into involuntary spasm. Second, the cough reflex will often try to expel the object.

Recognition

- The casualty may panic and become distressed.
- If standing, the casualty may stagger, become unsteady on their feet and may collapse.
- In the early stages the casualty's face may become flushed. In the later stages it may become pale, and cyanosis (blueness) may develop at the extremities.
- The casualty will be making distressed and perhaps violent efforts to breathe.
- The casualty's hands may grasp for the throat.
- The casualty's eyes may stare and begin to bulge.
- The casualty will often adopt a forward leaning posture. This helps the abdominal muscles to contract thus increasing the power of the cough reflex.

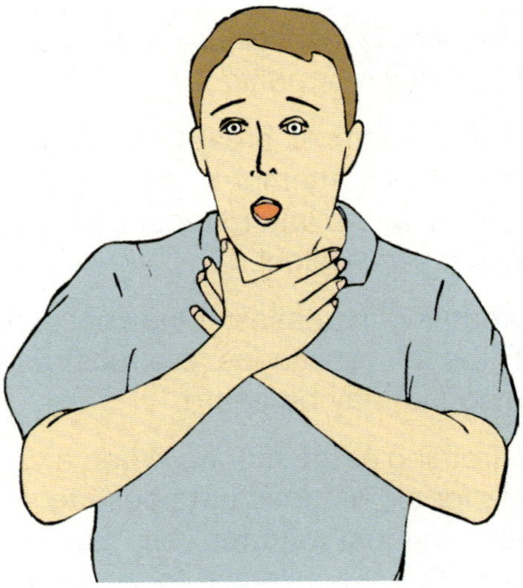

Fig.5. The Choking Casualty

Treatment

A situation where a person is choking can be very distressing for all concerned, but it is very important that treatment is administered in a calm and reassuring manner.

- If you are unaware of the history of the situation, ask the casualty if they are choking. They may confirm your suspicion with a nod.
- If possible, keep the casualty still (sitting or standing).
- Loosen any obvious tight, restrictive clothing such as a neck tie or belt.
- If the casualty is breathing, encourage him to continue coughing but do nothing else.
- If the casualty shows signs of becoming weak or stops breathing or coughing, leave him in the position in which you find him, remove any

obvious debris or loose false teeth from the mouth and carry out **back slaps.**

- Stand behind or to the side of the casualty, keeping them leaning well forward.
- Using the heel of the hand, give up to 5 sharp slaps between their shoulder blades.

Each slap may relieve the obstruction and it may not be necessary to give all five.

During the process, watch carefully for the object being expelled onto the floor.

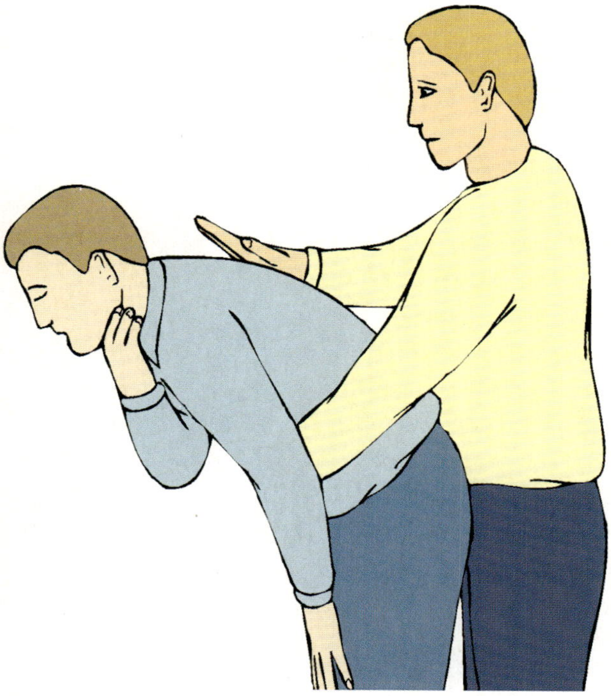

Fig.6. Administering Back Slaps

- If back slaps fail, **abdominal thrusts** may be tried.

The abdominal thrust is a very physical procedure to perform on a casualty and due to possible complications it should not be carried out on heavily pregnant women or on infants (see appendix H).

- Stand behind the casualty and put your arms around the casualty. Make a fist with one hand and place it against the casualty's upper abdomen (between the bottom of the breastbone and the navel) with the thumb innermost. Grasp the fist with the other hand.
- Pull sharply inwards and upwards. This has the effect of pushing the diaphragm upward and compressing the lungs. The obstruction should be expelled just like a cork from a bottle.

This abdominal thrust procedure may be attempted up to five times.

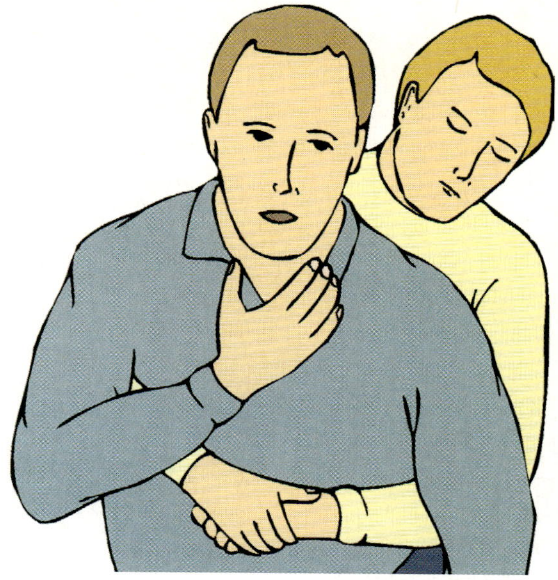

Fig.7. Administering Abdominal Thrusts

- If the obstruction is still not removed re-check the mouth for any obstruction which can be reached with a finger and continue alternating between five back slaps and five abdominal thrusts until either the object is removed or the casualty becomes unconscious.
- If the object is removed, put the casualty at rest and reassure them. Stay with the casualty and monitor them until breathing and skin colour return to normal.
- Any casualty on whom the abdominal thrust has been performed should be taken to hospital for further examination.

  If the throat of any casualty who has been choking remains sore, or shows any evidence of damage or bleeding, they should be taken to hospital for further examination.

To sum up choking for a conscious casualty:

- encourage to cough.
- give 5 back slaps.
- give 5 abdominal thrusts.
- repeat 5 slaps and 5 thrusts as necessary.

The Unconscious Choking Casualty

If the object is not removed from the throat, it may lead to unconsciousness.

Unconsciousness may result in relaxation of the muscles around the larynx (voicebox) and allow air to pass down into the lungs:

- Call for an ambulance.
- Carry out ABC (section 7) and try to give 2 effective rescue breaths.

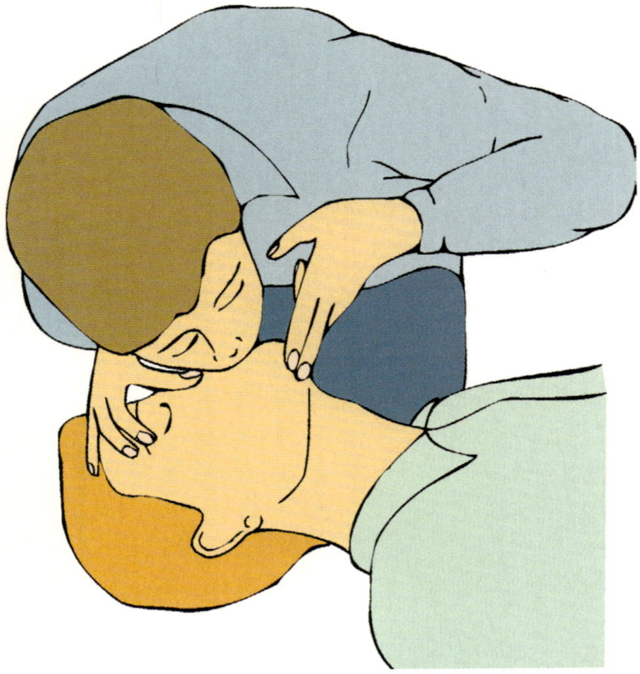

Fig.8. Rescue Breaths – Unconscious Choking Casualty

- If effective breaths **can** be achieved within 5 attempts, check for signs of a circulation (section 7) and start chest compressions and/or rescue breaths, as appropriate.
- If effective breaths **cannot** be achieved within 5 attempts, start chest compressions **immediately** to relieve the obstruction – do not check for signs of a circulation (it wastes time).
- After 15 compressions, check the mouth for any obstruction and then attempt further rescue breaths.

Continue to give cycles of 15 compressions followed by attempts at rescue breaths. If at any time effective breaths **can** be achieved:

- check for signs of a circulation.
- continue chest compressions and/or rescue breaths, as appropriate.

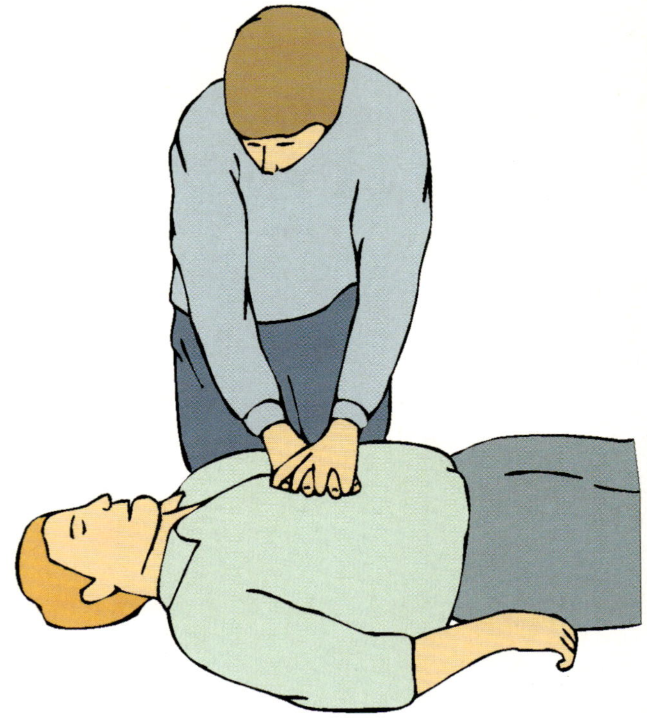

Fig.9. Chest Compressions – Unconscious Choking Casualty

To sum up choking for an unconscious casualty:

- carry out A and B of ABC.
- if breaths achieved, do C of ABC.
- do chest compressions or rescue breaths, as appropriate.
- if breaths not achieved, do NOT do C of ABC.
- do 15 compressions and 2 breaths.
- repeat as necessary.

Test Your Knowledge

1) What is the correct sequence for someone who has food stuck in his throat (please tick one):

   a) encourage to cough, 5 backslaps between shoulder blades, 5 abdominal thrusts
   b) 5 backslaps between shoulder blades, encourage to cough, 5 abdominal thrusts
   c) 5 backslaps between shoulder blades, 5 abdominal thrusts, encourage to cough
   d) 5 abdominal thrusts, encourage to cough, 5 backslaps between shoulder blades

2) What may prevent air getting through to the casualty's lungs during mouth-to-mouth?
   ....

3) If someone is choking and becomes unconscious and non-breathing, is it worth giving rescue breaths? ....

   Give a reason for your answer..

Emergency Diagnosis

Assessing the general condition of a casualty is the cornerstone of effective management. Incorrect diagnosis leads to incorrect treatment.

Before any treatment can commence, a diagnosis must be made to ascertain the general condition of the casualty. It is essential (and logical) that the most life-threatening conditions are found and treated first.

If the condition of a conscious casualty deteriorates, they will eventually become unconscious which causes voluntary muscles in the body to relax.

If an already unconscious casualty continues to deteriorate, the involuntary muscles of the body will stop working. Involuntary muscles are controlled subconsciously, that is to say a person does not have to think about their movement for the movement to occur. Examples of involuntary muscles are the diaphragm and the heart muscle. Just imagine how difficult life would be if you had to consciously think about it for your breathing and heart beat to occur!

The first group of involuntary muscles to stop functioning after unconsciousness are those concerned with breathing, i.e. the diaphragm and the intercostals. Stoppage of breathing is referred to as Respiratory Arrest.

If a non-breathing casualty should continue to deteriorate, the next group of involuntary muscles which will stop working are those of the heart. Stoppage of the heart is referred to as Cardiac Arrest.

The graph shows the possible path of deterioration of a casualty from 100% health down to death. As you can see, it is only a matter of minutes before unconsciousness, respiratory and cardiac arrest occur.

Every casualty who a first aider would need to treat will fall into one of the four different diagnosis areas or zones. Emergency Diagnosis is the procedure undertaken to ascertain which zone a casualty is presently in.

In this graph format, it is easy to see that generally a zone 2 casualty is worse than a zone 1 casualty. A zone 3 is worse than a zone 2 and so on. The worst possible general condition a casualty can be in, regardless of cause, is cardiac arrest.

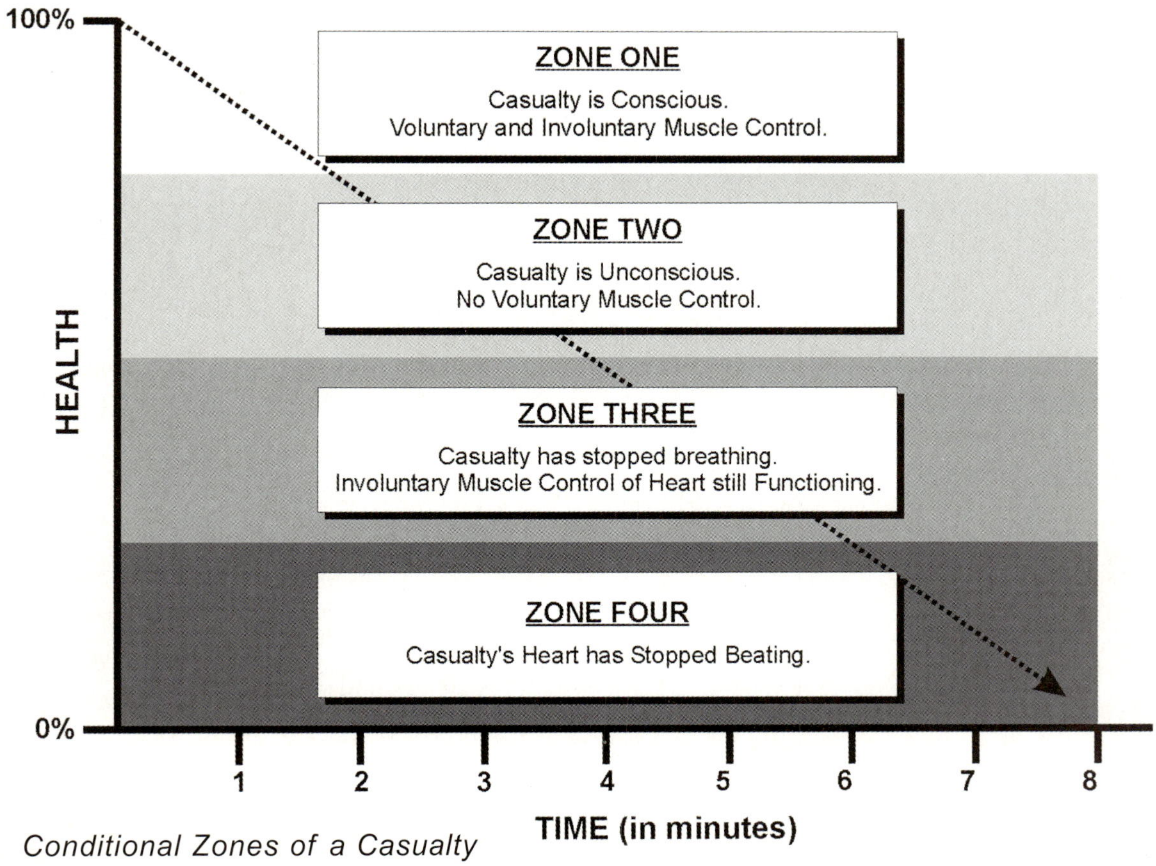

Fig.10. Conditional Zones of a Casualty

PRIMARY SURVEY

D Ensure there is no **Danger** to yourself or the casualty.

R Check for a **Response** from the casualty. Place your hands on the casualty's shoulders and gently shake them. At the same time loudly state a simple command such as "open your eyes" to determine if the casualty is conscious or unconscious (zone 1 or zone 2). If there is no response, shout for help in the local vicinity and proceed to Airway.

A If no response, clear and open the casualty's **Airway**.

When a person is unconscious, the voluntary muscles of the body relax, and the body will become generally limp and floppy. The tongue is a voluntary muscle and just like the arms and legs will relax. When the tongue relaxes it falls onto the back of the throat and causes an obstruction, thus closing the airway off.

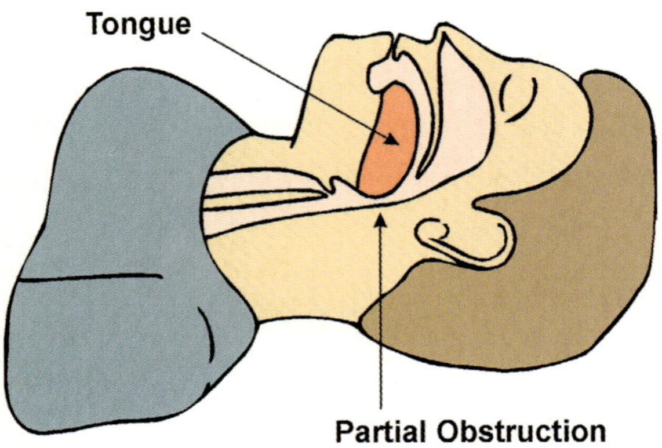

Fig.11. Closed Airway

As well as the tongue, there may also be foreign material or other obstructions inside the mouth such as dentures, broken teeth, chewing gum, saliva or vomit.

Obstruction of the airway due to the relaxed tongue is a major cause of death in the unconscious casualty and this problem must be dealt with immediately.

Opening the Airway

This is achieved by using the **head tilt - chin lift** procedure.

Inside the mouth, the tongue is connected to the jaw and if the chin is lifted upward, it will lift the tongue off the back of the throat. At the same time as the chin is lifted, the casualty's head should be tilted gently backward.

- Place the palm of one hand on the casualty's forehead, and gently tilt the casualty's head back. If there is an obvious visible obstruction inside the mouth, remove it. Lift the chin. If you suspect (due to the history of the accident) that the casualty may have head or neck injury, it is important that the movement is carried out slowly and carefully and only so far as to open the airway and not so far as to make any possible neck injury worse.
- Place two fingers of the other hand onto the bony prominence at the front of the casualty's chin. Do not press on the soft tissue under the chin as this will further obstruct the airway by pressing the tongue against the roof of the mouth.

Do not over extend or apply force to the neck when performing this technique. If you meet resistance to the head tilt, it usually indicates that the head is already well back. Continued tilting may cause further injury to the casualty.

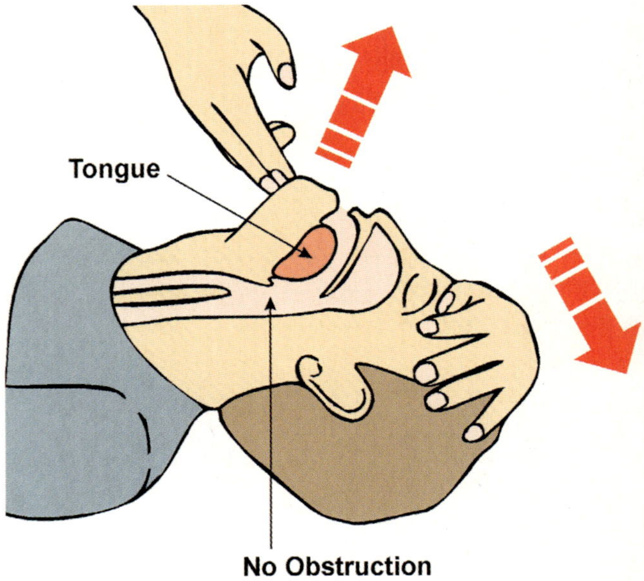

Fig.12. Opening the Airway

Removal of foreign objects from the mouth is best performed using the **finger sweep** technique.

- Insert your index finger into the casualty's mouth and sweep around the mouth in an attempt to hook the finger underneath the object and scoop it out.

  Do not use your fingers to feel blindly around the back of the throat.

  If an object is lodged firmly at the back of the throat, do not attempt to remove it with the finger sweep. Follow the procedures detailed for choking in an unconscious casualty (Page 6.2).

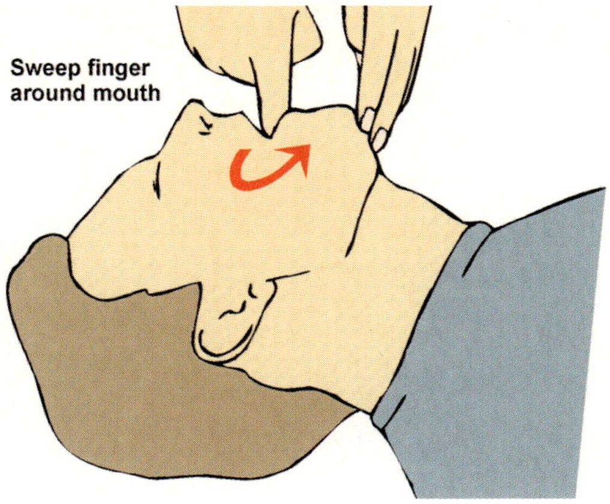

Fig.13. Clearing an Obstruction

B Keeping the-airway open, assess if the casualty is **Breathing** normally (more than the occasional gasp) by:

- Looking down the chest for any sign of movement.
- Listening for breathing sounds at the mouth.
- Feeling (with your cheek) for warm air being exhaled.

Look, listen and feel for no more than 10 seconds before deciding that normal breathing is absent.

If the casualty is breathing (more than an occasional gasp), treat as for the unconscious casualty (see section 9).

If the casualty is not breathing, send a bystander or helper for an ambulance and tell them to say that the casualty is not breathing. This specific information will help the ambulance service prioritise the call.

It is a fair assumption that by now, if the casualty is not breathing, the amount of oxygen in their blood will be down to a dangerously low level. It is therefore necessary at this stage to supply the casualty with oxygen by giving two effective breaths of artificial ventilation (see section 8).

C Assess if the casualty has **Circulation**. Look, listen and feel for normal breathing, coughing, movement, or any other signs of life. Assessment for circulation should take no more than 10 seconds.

If you are confident that the casualty has circulation, continue artificial ventilation and monitor the circulation every one minute.

If the casualty is not breathing and there are no signs of circulation (or you are at all unsure), chest compressions combined with artificial ventilation of the casualty's lungs will be necessary (see section 8).

When Do I Call for an Ambulance?

It is essential that professional help is called quickly if a casualty is not breathing. Therefore, if there is a bystander or helper at the scene, send them to call for an ambulance as soon as you know that the casualty is unresponsive and is not breathing.

If you are alone and the casualty is not breathing:

- If the likely cause of unconsciousness is:
  - **A**lcohol or
  - **D**rug intoxication;
  - **D**rowning; or if it is an
  - **I**nfant or child; or
  - **C**hoking; or
  - **T**rauma

give artificial ventilation (see Appendix H•1 and section 8) and assess for signs of circulation (as above). Resuscitate the casualty with artificial ventilation and if appropriate with chest compressions for one minute, then leave the casualty to call for an ambulance. On return to the casualty, recheck A.B.C. and continue resuscitation as necessary (see section 8).

- If the likely cause of unconsciousness is not as above, the first aider should assume that the casualty has a heart problem and go to call for an ambulance immediately it has been established that the casualty is not breathing. On return to the casualty, recheck A.B.C. and begin resuscitation as necessary (see section 8).

As HSE recommends that any first aider working regularly alone has the means to summon help in an emergency, it is unlikely that a first aider should need to leave any casualty.

Test Your Knowledge

1) If you are entirely alone with a non-breathing casualty, state the instances where you would give CPR for a minute before going to telephone for an ambulance:

a) Alcohol/ drugs .... b) chocking ....

c) children .... d) trauma ....

e) drowning .... f) ....

Resuscitation

The ability to take over for another person's breathing and circulation by artificial means are essential skills for all first aiders.

Resuscitation is the act of restoring function to the circulatory and/or respiratory systems when, for whatever reason, they have stopped.

Reasons why a person's breathing and circulation may stop are numerous, but the most common reasons include:

- Heart attack.
- Electric shock.
- Head injury.
- Poisoning, including drugs.
- Drowning.
- Blood loss leading to shock.

Stoppage of breathing and circulation is very serious, and quick diagnosis and treatment is essential.

Stoppage of Breathing

Stoppage of breathing is often referred to as respiratory arrest.

Diagnosis

Carry out the emergency diagnosis procedure (see section 7).

- Assess **Danger** (ensure safety).
- Assess **Response** (gently shake the casualty and shout for help in the local vicinity).
- Assess **Airway** (head tilt - chin lift).
- Assess **Breathing** (look, listen and feel).
- Assess **Circulation.**

Artificial Ventilation (Rescue Breathing).

If the casualty is not breathing normally, it is necessary to supply their body with oxygen by artificially ventilating their lungs (rescue breathing). The commonest form of rescue breathing used by first aiders is called mouth-to-mouth ventilation.

- If a bystander is available at the scene, send them for an ambulance as soon as you know that the casualty is not breathing.

- Turn the casualty onto their back if they are not already in this position.
- Give two effective breaths of mouth-to-mouth ventilation, each of which makes the chest rise:
    - Ensure head tilt. Remove any visible obstruction from the casualty's mouth including dislodged dentures, but leave well-fitting dentures in place. Lift the chin.

      Pinch the soft part of the casualty's nose closed with the index finger and thumb of the hand which is on their forehead.
    - Open the casualty's mouth a little but maintain chin lift. Take a deep breath and place your lips around their mouth, making sure that you have a good seal.
    - Blow steadily into their mouth over about 1 to 2 seconds, watching for their chest rising, as in normal breathing (in an adult, this usually requires 700-1000 ml of air). Be careful not to over-inflate the lungs as this may cause more problems.
    - Maintaining head tilt and chin lift, take your mouth away from the casualty and watch for their chest to fall as the air comes out.

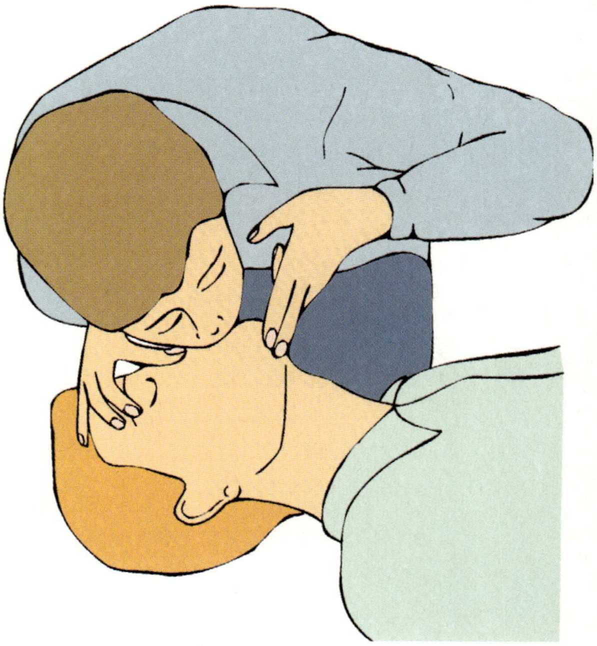

Fig.14. Rescue Breathing

- Take another breath and repeat the sequence.
- If you have difficulty in achieving an effective breath:

- Re-check the casualty's mouth and remove any visible obstruction.
- Re-check that there is adequate head tilt and chin lift.
- Make up to five attempts in all to achieve two effective breaths.

Even if unsuccessful, move on to assessment of circulation.

● Assess **Circulation**

(Assessment of the carotid pulse is time-consuming and often unrealiable. Performing a pulse check as a sign of cardiac arrest is no longer recommended for lay first-aiders.)

Look, listen and feel for normal breathing, coughing, or movement by the victim.

Take no more than 10 seconds to do this.

● If you are confident that you can detect signs of circulation within 10 seconds:

Continue rescue breathing, at a rate of one breath every six seconds, if necessary, until the casualty starts breathing on their own.

About every 10 breaths (or every one minute) recheck for signs of circulation. Take no more than 10 seconds each time.

● If the casualty begins to breathe normally on their own but remains unconscious, treat as for the unconscious casualty (see section 9).

● If there are no signs of circulation or if you are at all unsure, start chest compressions.

(Health care providers should still perform a pulse check as a sign of cardiac arrest and first aiders can still use a pulse check for monitoring the condition of an unconscious casualty as part of a top-to-toe survey.)

Stoppage of Circulation

Stoppage of circulation is often referred to as cardiac arrest. In cases of cardiac arrest, it is necessary to provide artificial circulation of the casualty's blood. The commonest method of providing artificial circulation is called chest compressions.

This is a very physical procedure in which firm pressure is applied to the casualty's chest with the intention of compressing the heart and pumping blood around the body.

Chest Compressions

● Locate the lower half of the casualty's breastbone (sternum):

- Using your index and middle fingers, identify the lower rib margin. Keeping your fingers together, slide them upwards to the point where the ribs join the sternum. With the middle finger on this point, place your index finger on the sternum.
- Slide the heel of your other hand down the sternum until it reaches your index finger; this should be the middle of the lower half of the sternum.
- Place the heel of the other hand on top of the first.
- Interlock the fingers of both hands and lift them to ensure that pressure is not applied to the casualty's ribs. Do not apply any pressure over the upper abdomen or bottom tip of the sternum.

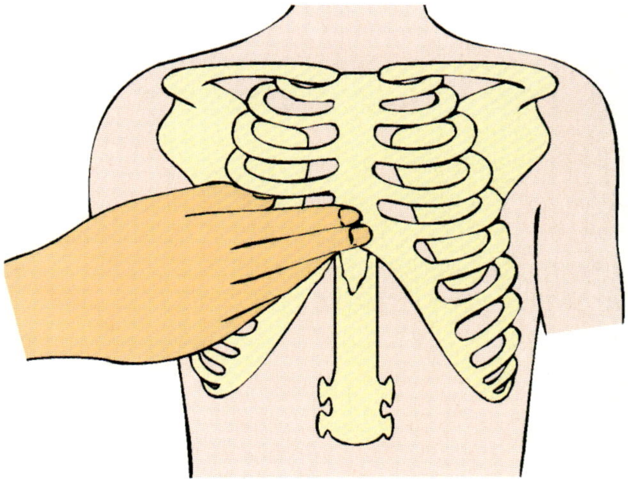

Fig.15. Compression Point

● Position yourself vertically above the casualty's chest and with your arms straight, press down on the sternum to depress it between 4-5cm (1½ to 2 inches).

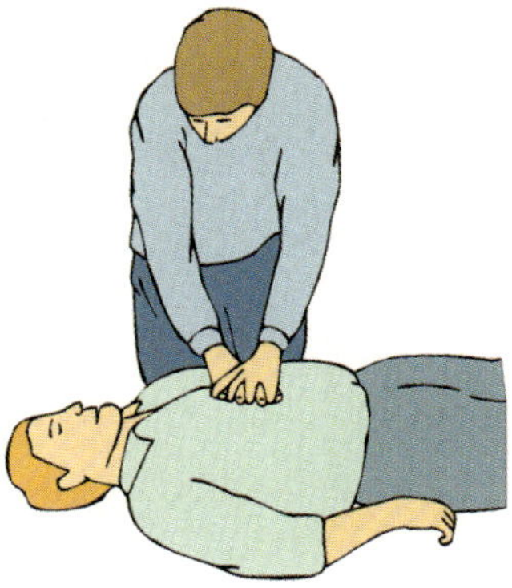

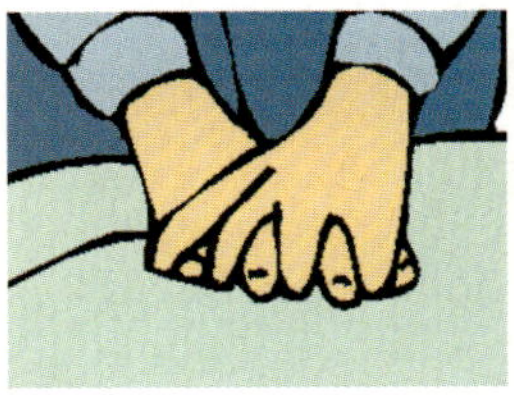

Interlock fingers.

Fig.16. Performing Chest Compressions

- Release the pressure, without losing contact between the hand and sternum, then repeat at a rate of 100 times a minute (a little less than two compressions a second). Compression and release should take an equal amount of time.

- Combine rescue breathing and chest compression:

- After 15 compressions, tilt the head, lift the chin and give two effective breaths.

  Return your hands without delay to the correct position on the sternum and give 15 further compressions, continuing breaths and compressions at a ratio of 2 to 15.

- Continue resuscitation until:
  - The ambulance arrives.
  - You become exhausted.
  - The casualty shows signs of life.

Only stop to recheck for signs of a circulation if the victim makes a movement or takes a spontaneous breath; otherwise, resuscitation should not be interrupted. If the casualty should at any point show signs of life or a return of circulation, eg movement, breathing, swallowing, coughing, etc, reassess for signs of a circulation. If you are confident that you can detect signs of circulation, stop performing chest compressions and continue rescue breathing at a rate of one ventilation every six seconds and re-check circulation every one minute.

As HSE recommends that any first aider working regularly alone has the means to summon help in an emergency, it is unlikely that a first aider should need to leave any casualty.

When Do I Call for an Ambulance?

It is essential that professional help is called quickly if a casualty is not breathing. Therefore, if there is a bystander or helper at the scene, send them to call for an ambulance as soon as you know that the casualty is unresponsive and is not breathing.

If you are alone and the casualty is not breathing:

- If the likely cause of unconsciousness is,

  Alcohol or
  Drug intoxication**;**
  Drowning; or if it is an
  Infant or child; or
  Choking; or
  Trauma

  give the two breaths of artificial ventilation and assess for signs of circulation (as above). Resuscitate the casualty with artificial ventilation and if appropriate with chest compressions for one minute, then leave the casualty to call for help. On return to the casualty, recheck A.B.C. and continue resuscitation as necessary.

- If the likely cause of unconsciousness is not as above, the first aider should assume that the casualty has a heart problem and go for help immediately it has been established that the casualty is not breathing. On return to the casualty, recheck A.B.C. and begin resuscitation as necessary.

Test Your Knowledge

1) You are attending an adult casualty who has just collapsed in front of you. There are no injuries. You find that they are not breathing and have no pulse. You are on your own. What immediate action should you take (please tick one answer):

   a) Leave the casualty and 'phone for an ambulance before commencing resuscitation.
   b) Commence resuscitation for a minute before 'phoning for an ambulance.
   c) Carry out resuscitation until help arrives.
   d) Place them into the recovery position and wait for someone else to arrive.

2) You are dealing with an unconscious adult casualty who has just been struck on the head by a falling scaffold pole. After checking that the airway is clear and open, you find that he is not breathing. You are on your own. What immediate action will you take (please tick one answer):

   a) Leave the casualty and 'phone for an ambulance before commencing resuscitation.
   b) Commence resuscitation for a minute before 'phoning for an ambulance.
   c) Carry out resuscitation until help arrives.
   d) Place them into the recovery position and wait for someone else to arrive.

3) How would you decide whether a casualty had stopped breathing?

   a) .... b) .... c) ....

4) How would you resuscitate someone who was bleeding from the mouth?

   ....

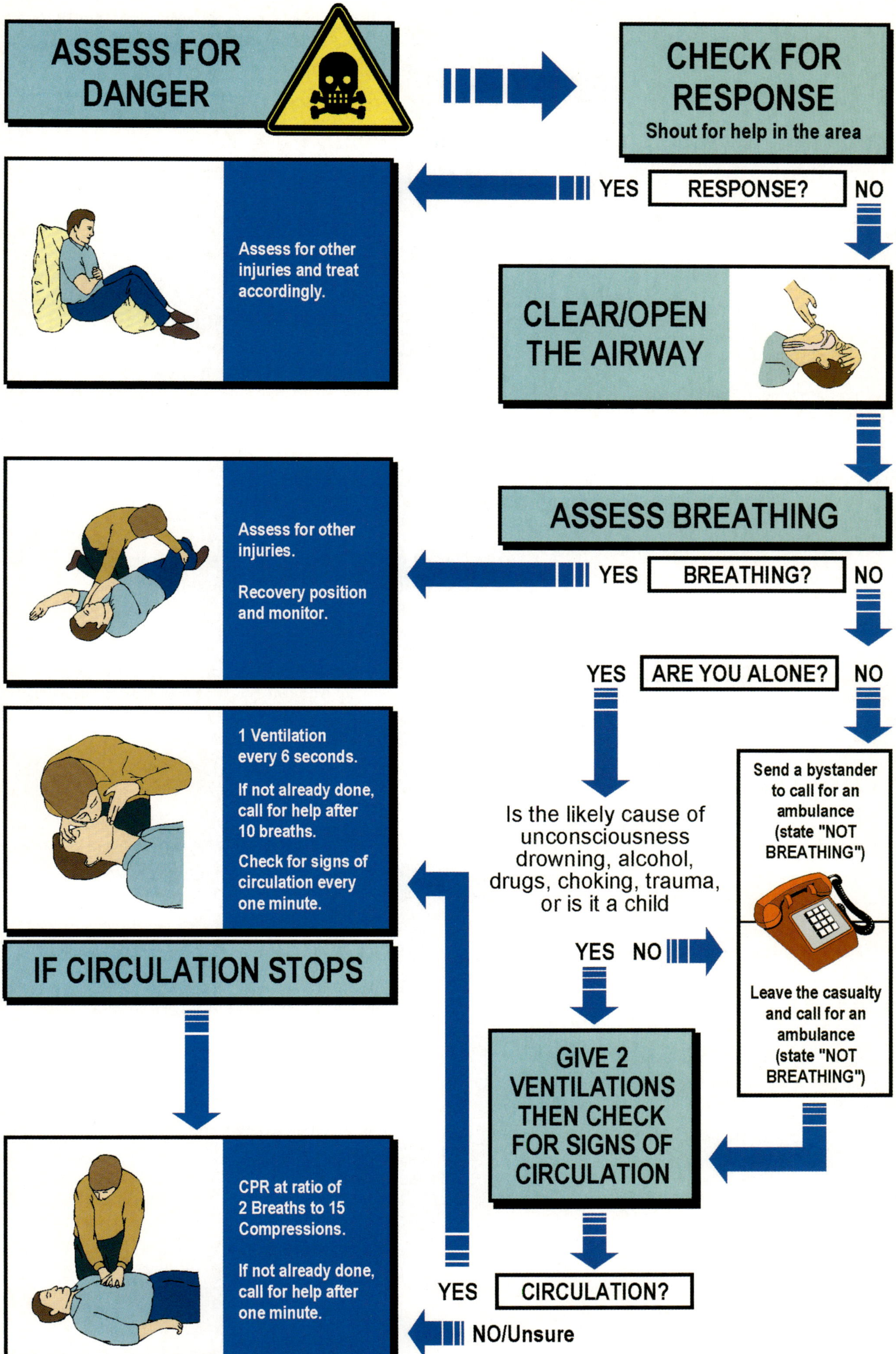

Fig.17. Resuscitation Flow Chart

The Unconscious Casualty

Unconsciousness can be a consequence of many injuries and sudden illnesses. The ability to deal promptly and effectively with an unconscious casualty is of great importance to all first aiders

Unconsciousness is defined as an interruption in the normal activity of the brain. The brain is a very complex organ, in fact so complex that even today very little is known and understood about how it manages to perform so many intricate and precise tasks. The brain is responsible for the control and co-ordination of nearly all body functions and, like the master processing chip inside a computer, if it becomes damaged the whole system may crash.

Situated within the protective confines of the skull, the brain is further protected by layers of tissue called meninges which completely surround it and its connecting link with the body, the spinal cord. Further protection is provided by a layer of fluid which is situated between two layers of the meninges, called cerebro-spinal fluid, which acts as a shock absorber.

Although reasonably well-protected, the cells of the brain are so delicate they are still very vulnerable to damage, be it temporary or permanent.

Common Causes of Unconsciousness

There are many individual causes of unconsciousness, but in general there are three main reasons why the normal functioning of the brain could be interrupted: physical damage to brain tissue caused by a head injury or stroke; chemical damage to brain tissue caused by increased levels of toxin or chemical substances in the blood stream; and lack of oxygen to brain tissue caused by asphyxiation or blood loss.

There are ten main common causes of unconsciousness. **F**ainting, **I**nfections, **S**troke, **H**ead injury, **S**hock, **H**eart attack, **A**sphyxia, **P**oisoning, **E**pilepsy and **D**iabetes. (F.I.S.H. S.H.A.P.E.D)

1. Fainting

This usually occurs when the oxygen supply to the brain is reduced. There are many things which could stimulate this such as lack of physical activity, and a warm, stuffy environment, but perhaps the commonest cause is emotional distress.

Most people have experienced some degree of overwhelming emotional distress in their lives, such as news of a bereavement, a good telling off by the boss at work or just reading their recent council tax bill. When subject to overwhelming emotional distress the body has a particular way of dealing with it. It is an involuntary or automatic response called the 'fight or flight syndrome' where the body quickly releases large amounts of chemical substances (one of which is called adrenalin) into the body tissues. These chemical substances, along with nervous impulses, cause a wide variety of physical reactions to occur inside the body, such as an increase in the blood pressure, an increase in heart and breathing rates, a reduction in blood flow to the skin and guts and the stimulation of the sweating mechanism.

If a person is in an upright posture when this occurs, the forces of gravity prevent much of the blood returning up to the heart and head. This brief lack of blood and oxygen to the brain causes dizziness and eventually interrupts brain activity so much that unconsciousness can result.

This mild form of unconsciousness associated with a simple faint is usually brief and treatment involves returning blood flow and oxygen supply to the brain.

- Lay the casualty down on their back.
- Keep the airway open and clear and loosen any tight or restrictive clothing.
- Elevate their legs to improve the return of blood to the top half of the body.

If recovery is swift, no further treatment is usually required. If the faint or dizzy spell is persistent or occurs on a frequent basis, the casualty should be advised to see a doctor at the earliest possible opportunity. If the unconsciousness lasts for more than just a few minutes, place the casualty in the recovery position and call for an ambulance.

2. Infections

When the body is invaded by microscopic organisms such as viruses and bacteria, it reacts in many different ways to fight off the infection, such as the production of antibodies and the raising of body temperature. If the infection is severe and spreads to the brain tissue, unconsciousness can result.

3. Stroke

Otherwise known as a cerebro-vascular accident (CVA), a stroke occurs when small blood vessels in the brain become obstructed (usually due to a blood clot). This obstruction will cause a reduction or absolute stoppage of blood supply to the brain tissue, resulting in oxygen deprivation and tissue death. Furthermore, pressure builds up behind the blockage in the blood vessel which causes it to distend and eventually rupture. The effects of a stroke depend primarily on how much, and which part, of the brain is affected, but in many cases it will interfere with the normal activity of the brain and result in unconsciousness (see appendix C).

4. Head Injuries

One of the most common causes of unconsciousness, but in many cases it is only temporary and reversible. The duration and depth of the resulting unconsciousness depends on the severity of the subsequent brain damage (see section 17).

5. Shock

There are many different types of shock. The body's reaction to overwhelming emotional circumstances is known as emotional or neurogenic shock (as described in fainting above). True or hypovolaemic shock develops when the body loses circulating fluid, such as blood. This would reduce blood pressure and oxygen supply to vital areas, thus causing an interference in the normal activity of the brain and unconsciousness (see section 11).

6. Heart Attack

This occurs when the heart muscle is starved of oxygen, usually due to a blockage in the arteries (coronary) which supply it with blood. If the muscle cells in the heart are starved of oxygen they will not function correctly and therefore the heart beat becomes weak and irregular. This lowers blood pressure and reduces blood flow to the brain (see appendix B).

7. Asphyxia

If the blood is unable to obtain sufficient oxygen for whatever reason, it will follow that there will be a reduction on the oxygen supply to the brain, eventually resulting in unconsciousness (see section 5).

8. Poisoning

When harmful substances enter the body they can easily work themselves into the blood stream which is a direct and unobstructed route to the vital organs, especially the brain (see section 19).

9. Epilepsy

Epilepsy is described as a tendency to experience repeated muscular contractions or convulsions which are due to an internal problem in the brain. There are many different types of epilepsy, each with its own particular traits and recognition points, but all types involve some degree of electrical disturbance in the brain, many of which cause some degree of unconsciousness (see appendix E).

10. Diabetes

This is a condition in which the body fails to regulate the amount of sugar (glucose) in the blood stream. If the blood sugar level rises or falls outside of certain parameters it can have a severe and adverse effect on the body, in particular brain activity (see appendix D).

Treatment of Unconsciousness

In most cases of unconsciousness, there is very little a first aider can do to reverse the primary cause, therefore general treatment revolves around the main problem associated with the unconsciousness itself - airway obstruction.

After performing the primary survey (unresponsive but breathing and pulse present):

1. Perform a Secondary Survey

This is a systematic and methodical assessment of the casualty's body to determine the presence or absence of injuries, and evidence of other important details relating to the casualty.

You should:

- Listen to the history of the accident and look for external clues
- if an accident, find out how it happened and the forces involved
- look for signs and symptoms
- examine the casualty

It is logical that in any examination of a casualty the most serious and life threatening injuries are found first. When carrying out the examination, the first aider should always bear in mind the cause and history of the accident which will have great significance on exactly where and what type of injuries the casualty may have sustained. For example, a casualty who has been subject to direct impact and violence to the body is much more likely to have sustained broken bones than a casualty who has collapsed due to overheating. A casualty who was subject to blast and fragmentation is much more likely to sustain open wounds than a casualty who has suffered an allergic reaction to an insect sting, and so on.

The examination will involve the use of the first aider's senses of touch, sight and smell and it is carried out in two stages.

Use both hands together to compare one side of the body to the other. Feel underneath clothing if necessary. Use the tips of your fingers where possible to increase sensitivity.
If necessary, remove or re-position any clothing which obstructs clear vision of the skin and body surface in areas where you suspect an injury to be present.

Put on a pair of protective examination gloves before commencing a top-to-toe examination of a casualty.

Stage 1

Check quickly but thoroughly all the way down the body (including the limbs) for any sign of serious bleeding. If serious bleeding is found, deal with it immediately.

Stage 2

Check the body again from the head to the feet for other injuries and any evidence relating to the possible cause of the unconsciousness.

- Head & Neck

  Feel for any deformity, swelling, lumps, and indentations.

  Look for any minor bleeding, bruising or deformities. Look for any liquid or blood leaking from the eyes, ears or nose.

  Look at the eyes to see if they are bloodshot.

  Look for a Medic-Alert or other talisman around the casualty's neck. This could give information on any medical condition which the casualty suffers from, such as epilepsy, diabetes or allergies.

  Smell the casualty's breath for alcohol or unusual smells such as acetone (like nail varnish remover).

- Shoulders

  Feel for any deformity and swelling, especially around the collar bones.

  Look for any minor bleeding and bruising.

- Chest

  Feel for any deformities.

  Look for any unnatural movement of the chest wall and for any minor bleeding.

- Abdomen

  Feel for any deformity or hard areas (which could indicate internal injury) and for any minor bleeding.

- Hips

  Feel for any deformity.

  Look for any minor bleeding.

  Look for any damp patches in the groin area which may indicate that the casualty has urinated.

  Remove any bulky or sharp objects from the casualty's pockets which may cause injury when rolling into the recovery position. Ensure that any objects which are removed are kept safe and passed on to the ambulance service when they arrive. If possible, put the objects into a container or envelope, label it with the casualty's details and have a second person witness that your actions were necessary and above-board.

- Arms & Hands

  Feel for any deformity or swelling.

  Look for any minor bleeding and for a Medic-Alert or other talisman around the wrist.

- Legs & Feet

  Feel for any deformity or swelling.

  Look for any minor bleeding, or dampness between the legs.

Exactly how long this check should take and how thorough it should be again depends primarily on the history. If a casualty has been subject to blast and fragmentation, the damage to the body could be extensive and therefore more time should be taken. If a casualty has only fainted, damage to the body would be minimal therefore less time would be taken. If the examination is lengthy, keep going back to check the airway and breathing every minute or so. It would be poor technique to spend ten minutes performing a thorough examination only to find out that the casualty stopped breathing eight minutes ago.

If any serious injuries are found during the examination, it may be necessary to treat them before further treatment for the unconsciousness continues. If this is so, keep a close watch on the airway and breathing throughout treatment.

0Warning key rings, bracelets and necklaces such as Medic-Alert and S.O.S. talisman provide details of medical information pertaining to the person carrying or wearing it. Commonest indications they give are for diabetes, epilepsy and allergies.

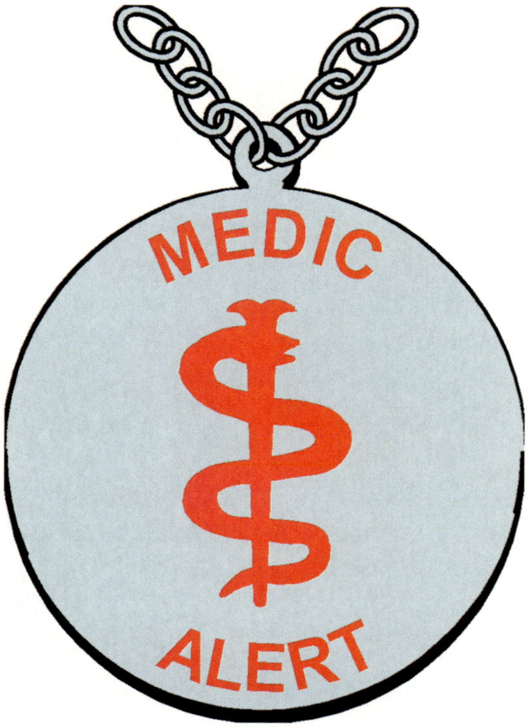

Fig.18. Medic-Alert

2. Place the Casualty in the Recovery Position

Without specialised equipment it can be very dangerous to leave an unconscious casualty laid on their back.

- Even with the airway extended, the tongue could still slightly close off the airway.
- If the casualty should suddenly vomit, it would cause airway obstruction and the vomit may be inhaled.
- Saliva which secretes into the mouth would drain to the back of the throat and be inhaled.

Bearing these factors in mind, unconscious casualties should be placed in a position which alleviates these potential problems - the Recovery Position.

There are many different variations of the recovery position, each with their own individual attributes and benefits. Regardless of which individual position is used, there are six specific criteria which should be observed.

- The position is as near true lateral position as possible with the head dependent to allow free drainage of fluid.
- The position should be stable.
- Any pressure on the chest which impairs breathing should be avoided.
- It should be possible to turn the casualty onto the side and return to the back easily and safely having particular regard to the possibility of a neck or spine injury.
- Good observation and access to the airway should be possible.
- The position itself should not give rise to any injury to the casualty.

To turn a casualty into the recovery position:

- Kneel next to the casualty and raise the arm which is nearest to you, out to the side. This ensures that the casualty will not roll on to the arm which could restrict breathing.

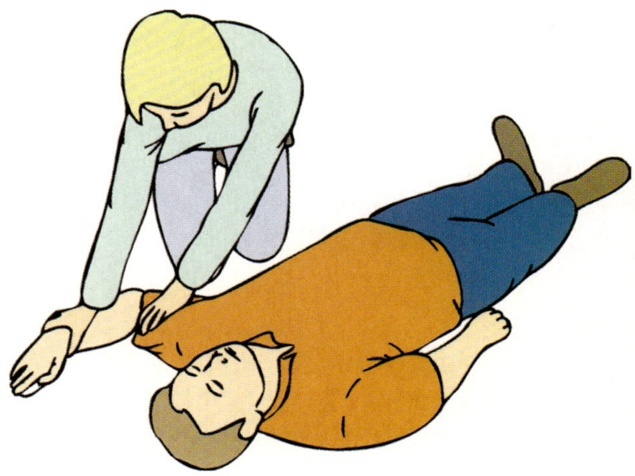

- Reach across the casualty, lift up their hand (palm-to-palm) and gently place the back of their hand against the side of their face. If the casualty is wearing a ring which could scratch their face, carefully turn it around so the sharp or bulky part is facing the palm.

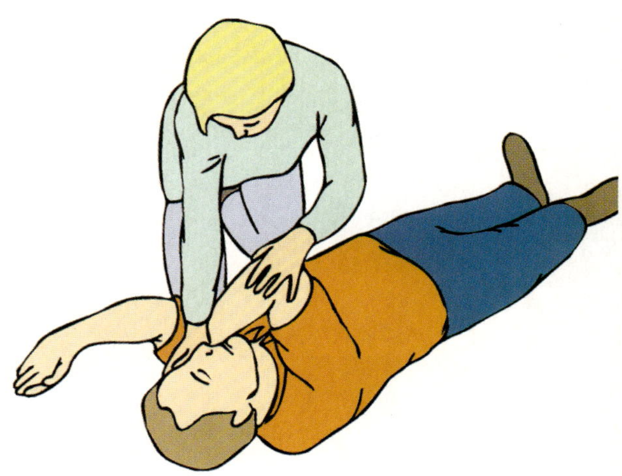

- Keeping this hand in position to support the head, lift the opposite knee with the other hand. The bent leg will now provide a lever with which to roll the casualty.

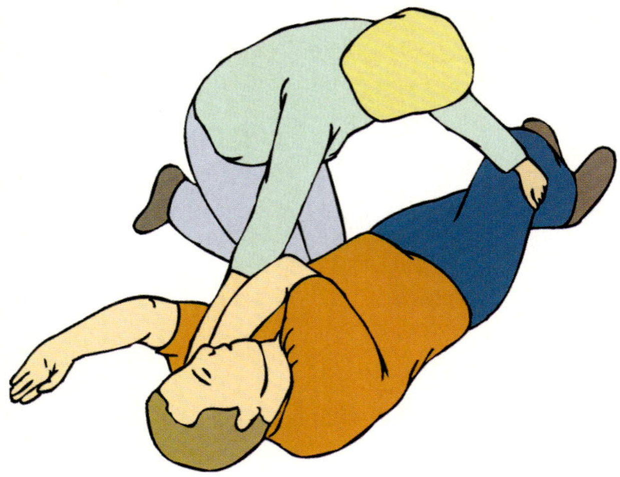

Fig.19. Turning a casualty into the Recovery Position

- Supporting the head with one hand, gently pull the knee towards you and the casualty will begin to turn. Allow the casualty to turn approximately three quarters of the way over onto their front. By now the knee on which you were pulling should be in contact with the floor.
- Gently remove your hand from underneath the cheek and allow the casualty's head to rest on the back of their hand. Gently tilt the head back to ensure the airway remains open and re-check breathing.
- Pull up on the knee of the upper leg so the hip and knee are bent at approximately right angles. This bent leg will stop the casualty rolling over completely onto their front.
- Check the circulation in the arm which passes under the casualty's body by feeling for the radial pulse at the wrist. If the pulse is absent or there is any sign that circulation into the arm is interrupted, slightly reposition the arm until normal circulation returns.
- If the casualty has to be kept in the recovery position for more than 30 minutes, if injuries permit they should be turned onto the opposite side - this relieves pressure on the circulation of the lower arm.

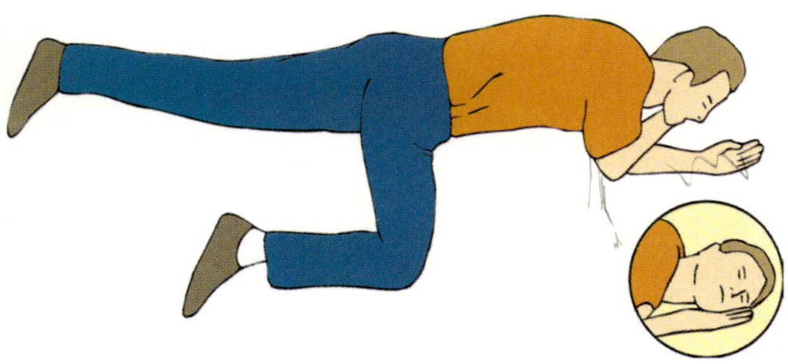

Fig.20. The Recovery Position

Modifying the Recovery Position

In some cases the unconscious casualty may already be lying on their front when you arrive on the scene. If this is so,

- Carry out the A.B.C. of emergency diagnosis.If the casualty is not breathing, they must be carefully turned onto their back for resuscitation.

If the casualty is breathing, it is unnecessary to turn them on to their back, just to turn them back on to their front. A modified recovery position can be achieved by simply and gently repositioning their limbs.

- Note which way the head is already turned and carefully move the hand on this side between the face and the ground. Ensure that the airway remains open.
- Bend and raise the knee on the same side. This will lift the casualty's abdomen and lower chest off the ground and allow for unrestricted breathing.
- Ensure the arm on the opposite side of the body is in a safe position and check the radial pulse to ensure that circulation is not impeded.

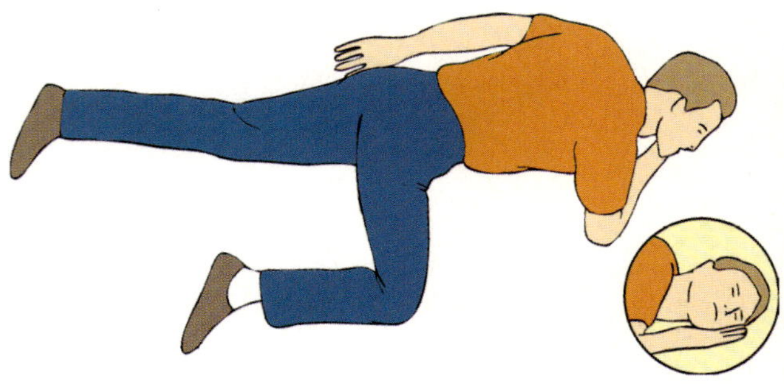

Fig.21. Modified Recovery Position

In some cases, the top-to-toe examination of the casualty may have discovered the presence of other injuries, in particular broken bones (fractures).

If you suspect fractures to the arms or legs, the position may again need to be modified to take account of the injury. Remember, nothing takes priority over the casualty's airway and breathing, but when modifying the position, try to move the injured area as little as possible.

The Spinal Injury Recovery Position

Perhaps the most daunting situation with an unconscious casualty is when spinal injuries are suspected. In many cases it may be impossible for the first aider to tell if the casualty's back or neck is injured. If the history and circumstances of the accident indicate that the casualty has been subject to violence or direct impact (such as a fall or being hit by a falling object), the golden rule is to always suspect that the spine may be damaged and to take this into account when rolling the casualty over.

Use the jaw thrust to maintain an airway in these casualties, unless they are vomiting or you need to leave them.

- Kneel behind the casualty's head.
- Place your hands on each side of the head with your fingertips at the angles of the jaw.
- Gently lift the jaw to open the airway.
- Take care not to tilt the casualty's head.

If vomiting or unconscious and you need to leave the casualty, use a recovery position:

- "normal" recovery position if you are alone
- if you have one helper, one person steadies the had and second person turns the casualty
- if you have two helpers, one person steadies the head, the second turns the casualty and the third helps to keep the back in alignment with the head
- if you have three or more helpers, use the log roll technique – remove spectacles and bulky objects in pockets.

Don't forget to "read the accident" – if there is a history of force to the body of any sort, always suspect spinal injuries. This includes any injury to the head.

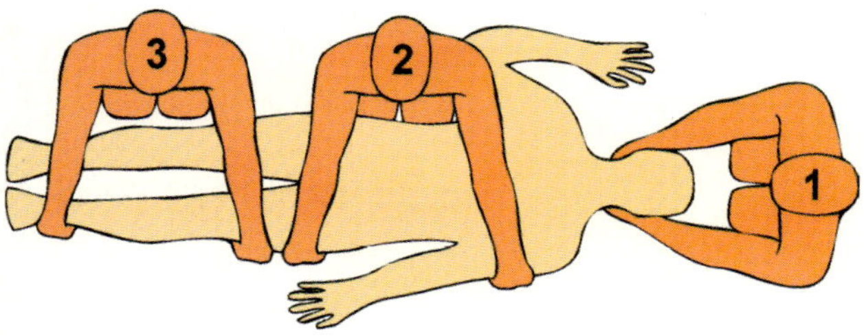

Fig.22. Positions for turning - Spinal Injury Recovery Position

- Person number 1 should call out the timing for the turn, e.g. ready... steady... turn. This will ensure that persons 2 and 3 start pulling at the same time.
- Persons 2 and 3 should now pull the casualty toward themselves, ensuring that they are pulling at the same speed to ensure the whole body remains straight. Person number 1 should ensure that as the body is turned, the nose remains constantly on the mid line of the body, thus not allowing the neck to twist or bend.

  The turning process should be slow enough to ensure the whole body is 'log rolled' 90 degrees until the casualty is laid on their side.
- Once over on their side, padding should be inserted between the ground and the casualty's lower cheek to ensure that the head does not fall, twisting the neck.

  The airway should be assessed and a check made to ensure there is no restriction on movement of the chest wall.

  Circulation in the lower arm should be checked for impediment by feeling the radial pulse.
- Padding should now be placed around the casualty to stabilise the position.

3. Perform a Head to Heel Examination

Now that the casualty has been turned over, a further examination for injuries should be carried out down the casualty's back.

The examination should look for open wounds, bleeding, swelling, deformity and discolouration of the skin. If clothing impedes visual inspection, it should be carefully adjusted or removed if necessary. If any injuries are found, treat accordingly.

4. Carry out Basic Observations

The casualty must now be monitored regularly for any sign of change in their condition. A written record should be made of the findings and passed on to the ambulance service when they arrive.

- **Information to Record**
  - A brief history of the accident, and if possible the personal details of the casualty such as name, address, age, etc.
  - The nature and approximate time of the accident.
  - Notes about any injuries found on the casualty, or any evidence which helps determine the cause of unconsciousness. Details of any medication which the casualty takes or allergies they have (if known).
  - Details of any treatment given.
- **Observations to Record**

There are five basic observations to record. Breathing, pulse, pupils, pallor and response.

  - Breathing. Note details of its rate, depth and regularity. Remember, the normal breathing rate for an adult at rest is 14 to 18 breaths per minute.
  - Pulse. Note details of its rate (speed), strength and regularity. Remember, the normal pulse rate for an adult at rest is 60 to 80 beats per minute.
  - Pupils. Note if they are equal in size and if they react to light. Irregular or fixed pupils often indicate that the brain is damaged in some way.

- Pallor. Note the colour of the casualty's skin. Is it pale, flushed, or normal? Look for blueness, especially at the extremities (cyanosis). Feel the temperature of the casualty's face. Is it warm, cold or normal?
- Level of response. This helps determine the depth of unconsciousness.

  A - Are they alert and opening their eyes spontaneously?

  V - Do they respond to your voice? Give them simple commands such as "open your eyes".

  P - Do they respond to painful stimuli? Gently pinch the very end of the casualty's ear lobe. Look for an automatic reflex such as a flinch of the eye, movement of the facial muscles or perhaps even a groan.

  U - Are they unresponsive to all stimuli?

You must only leave an unconscious casualty if it is absolutely necessary, e.g. when you are alone and have to go and call for an ambulance. If you must leave the casualty, ensure that they are in the recovery position before you leave. It may be necessary to place support behind the casualty to make the position more stable and ensure that they cannot roll over onto their back in your absence.

If at any time the casualty should stop breathing, gently but quickly roll them back onto their back and commence resuscitation as appropriate.

Test Your Knowledge

1) You are dealing with a casualty who is breathing but unconscious. There are no obvious injuries. You should now (please tick one answer):

   a) Go and phone for an ambulance.
   b) Fill out the accident report book.
   c) Place the casualty into the recovery position.
   d) Avoid moving them in case you make the condition worse.

2) From the list below, tick the four aspects that you consider to be the most important when dealing with an unconscious casualty:

   a) Keep the casualty warm
   b) Complete the accident book
   c) Place in the recovery position
   d) Phone for an ambulance
   e) Resuscitate if necessary
   f) Establish levels of responsiveness
   g) Carry out general body check/observations
   h) Maintain airway

3) You are dealing with a casualty who is breathing but unconscious.

   a) What position should you place the casualty in? ....
   b) Give two reasons why this position should be used.

      i ....
      ii ....

4) When dealing with an unconscious casualty, there are four levels of responsiveness. What are they?

   A ....V ....P ....U ....

Wounds and Bleeding

Bleeding is a very common type of injury and most first aiders in the workplace will at some point have to deal with an open wound.

Whenever blood vessels are punctured, split, torn, cut or severed, the blood inside will leak out. Exactly how much blood is lost from a wound depends largely on the type and size of blood vessels which have been damaged.

Types of Bleeding

1. Arterial Bleeding

The blood inside arteries is usually under a high degree of pressure so when an artery is damaged the resulting blood loss can be very serious. This type of bleeding can be very difficult to control, especially if large arteries are damaged.

In some cases of severe external bleeding, it is possible to see the blood from a damaged artery spurting from the wound in time with the heart beat. The majority of arteries in the body carry oxygenated blood which usually gives arterial bleeding a very bright red appearance.

2. Venous Bleeding

The blood inside veins is not usually under a high degree of pressure so when a vein is damaged the resulting blood loss is not as serious as that from a similar-sized artery. As the pressure is low, this type of bleeding is fairly easy to control. Again, due to the lower pressure, the blood from a vein will flow rather than spurt from the wound. The majority of veins carry de-oxygenated blood which usually gives a dark red appearance.

3. Capillary Bleeding

Bleeding from capillaries is not usually serious and control can be achieved with simple techniques.

In general, the higher the degree of blood pressure inside the blood vessel, the quicker the blood loss will be.

Minor Wounds

Minor wounds such as small cuts, scratches and grazes are common injuries but treatment is simple.

- Gently clean the wound with fresh tap water or, if water is not available, use an individually wrapped moist cleansing wipe from the first aid kit. When clean, dry the area with the gauze pad of a sterile dressing.
- Apply a suitably-sized adhesive dressing over the wound, ensuring that all the wound is covered and the adhesive element of the dressing does not come into contact with the wound itself.
- If a suitable adhesive dressing is not available, use a sterile wound dressing. The bleeding will usually stop quickly due to the natural clotting reaction of the blood

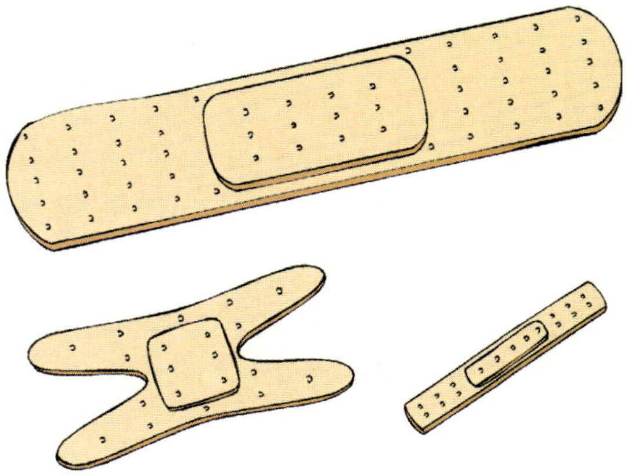

- Advise the casualty to watch out for signs of infection in the wound such as tenderness, swelling, reddening or pus oozing from the wound. Advise the casualty to see their doctor if infection becomes evident. In some cases, the casualty may need to have a tetanus injection following even the most minor wound. If there is a risk from tetanus and the casualty does not know if they are up to date with their immunisation, the casualty should again be advised to seek further medical aid from their doctor.

Advise the casualty to return to you if bleeding persists.

- Record the details in the accident book.

Major Wounds

There is no specific dividing line between what constitutes a minor wound and what constitutes a major wound, but in the context of most first aid treatments major wounds are generally classified as those which require more than just the application of a simple adhesive dressing, i.e. bleeding from arteries and veins. The casualty will need an ambulance.

There are three main elements to the treatment of major wounds. **R**est, **E**levation and **D**irect Pressure (R.E.D.)

1. Rest the Casualty

As already explained, the speed of blood loss from a wound will be directly proportional to the pressure of blood inside the damaged blood vessels, therefore factors which raise the blood pressure unnecessarily should be avoided. These include emotional distress and physical activity.

To overcome these factors, the casualty should be:

- allowed to adopt a comfortable resting position usually sitting down, although in cases where shock develops, laying down with the legs slightly elevated (see section 11);
- reassured as to the severity of the injury and the competence of the first aider.

2. Elevate the Wound

If the wound is supported at a level above that of the heart, blood will have to travel upwards to reach the wound. The increased gravitational effect will help reduce the blood flow (and pressure) to the wound. If elevation of the wound is not possible due to the nature or location of the wound, try at least to get the wound level with the heart and not below it.

If there is a suspected broken bone in the area of the wound (open fracture), ensure that the bone is completely immobilised before elevation otherwise movement of the bone ends will cause more damage to the surrounding tissue and make the bleeding worse. If in doubt, do not elevate open fractures.

3. Apply Direct Pressure

This is the main principle in the control of bleeding. The application of counter pressure on the wound will reduce the pressure and speed at which blood exits, just like putting your thumb over the end of a hose pipe.

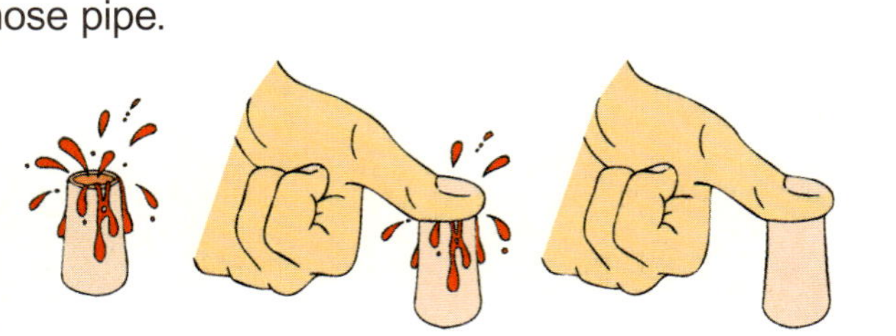

Fig.23. The Principle of Counter Pressure

Exactly how much counter pressure is required will be entirely dependent on the pressure at which the blood comes out of the damaged blood vessels. Arterial bleeding often requires a high degree of counter pressure to stop the blood flow.

Before applying a pressure dressing, examine the wound for any embedded objects. If an object is embedded in the wound e.g. metal or glass, an alternative method of application will be necessary (see Embedded Objects).

Pressure should be applied to an open wound using a sterile wound dressing. Wound dressings come in a huge variety of shapes and sizes and most first aid kits contain a good selection. The Health and Safety Executive issue guidance to employers which recommends that two approximate sizes of wound dressing should be made available, 12cm x 12cm and 18cm x 18cm. Further to this, wound dressings should be sterile, individually wrapped and unmedicated.

The chosen dressing should, if possible, be large enough to cover the entire wound. If the wound is very large, it may take multiple dressings to ensure complete coverage.

There are many different methods of applying wound dressings, but regardless of which method is used, the following principles must apply:

- carefully remove or cut away all clothing around the wound. A dressing should not be used over the top of clothing as this may reduce its effect;
- sterility of the dressing should be maintained. Try not to touch the face of the sterile pad when unwrapping and applying the dressing;
- the pad of the dressing should be placed in a central position over the wound and all the wound should be covered;
- the tails should be wrapped around without twisting or screwing up. This will ensure that the tails do not dig in and, in the case of a limb, will reduce the chances of circulation impediment;
- when applied, the tails should cover all the pad and the pressure should be evenly distributed across all the pad. If pressure is only applied in the middle, blood will seep out from the sides;
- the tail ends should be secured in position to prevent them from unwrapping. This is usually achieved by tying a knot or using a safety pin from the first aid kit;

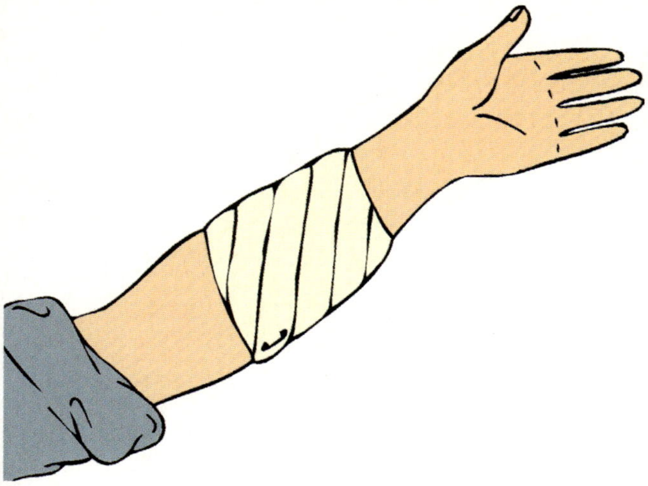

Fig.24. Pressure Dressing

- in cases of bandages to the limbs, check the circulation in the limb once the bandage is applied. If the bandage is too tight it could cut off the circulation, making the limb go pale and cold. The casualty may also begin to sense a numbness or tingling sensation in the limb. If circulation is impeded, the dressing may have to be loosened slightly;
- monitor the dressing to ensure that the bleeding is controlled;
- if one dressing is insufficient to control the bleeding, blood will eventually seep through.

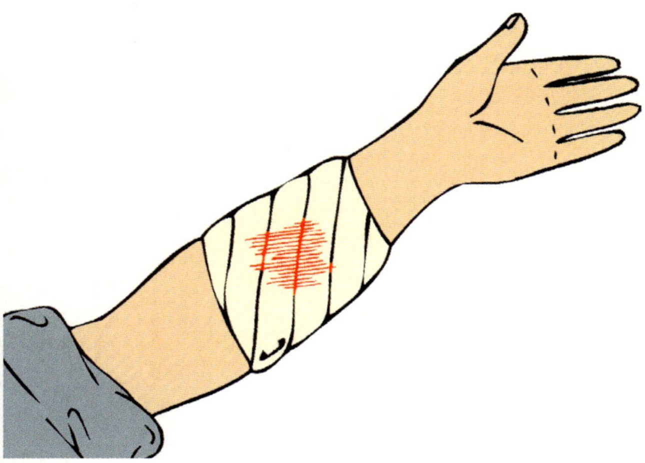

If this occurs, apply a second dressing over the top of the first, in exactly the same way. Do not remove the initial dressing. The combined pressure from two pressure bandages may be enough to stop the bleeding;

Soggy dressings after treating bleeding

The first aider should, if blood seeps through two dressings, remove them and apply a new one. (If the original dressing was applied accurately to the point of bleeding with appropriate pressure – firm enough to stop bleeding but not so firm as to cut off circulation – this should not be necessary.)

Indirect Pressure (Pressure Points)

In extreme cases, blood may seep through the third pressure bandage. A fourth dressing over the top of the third is unlikely to add any more significant pressure, therefore the only course of action remaining is to reduce the blood flow to the wound.

As explained in section 4, arteries carry blood to all parts of the body. The principle of indirect pressure is to apply pressure not to the wound, but to the artery which supplies the wound with blood. Indirect pressure to control bleeding is applied on an artery at a point where it passes over a bone - a 'pressure point'.

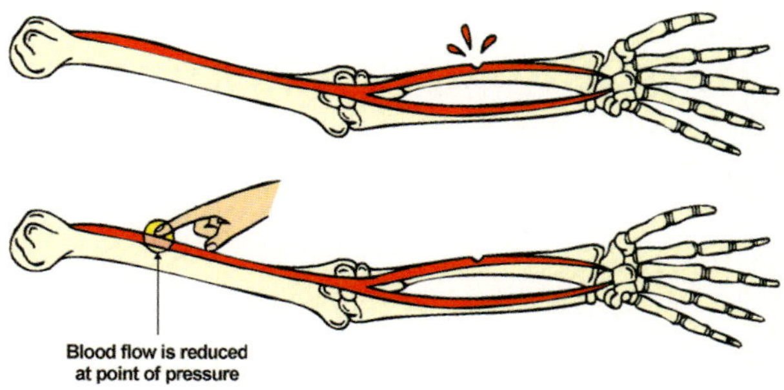

Fig.25. The Principle of Indirect Pressure (Pressure Points)

Pressure points can be found all over the body but first aid is generally limited to the use of two. The brachial pressure point in the upper arm and the femoral pressure point in the groin.

1. The Brachial Pressure Point

The brachial pressure point can be located on the brachial artery in the upper arm. The brachial artery lies between the upper arm muscle (biceps) and the upper arm bone (humerus). If pressure is applied in the correct place, the first aider should be able to feel the brachial pulse.

Pressure is applied by gripping around the upper arm, with the finger tips pressing directly on the artery. In most cases it is necessary to remove any clothing from the upper arm. Applying pressure over clothing can make the technique very difficult.

2. The Femoral Pressure Point

The femoral pressure point can be located on the femoral artery in the upper leg. The femoral artery runs from the front of the groin, down the inner aspect of the upper leg and ends at the back of the knee. The artery comes closest to the surface of the body at the front of the groin. If pressure is applied in the correct place, the first aider should be able to feel the femoral pulse.

Pressure is applied by gripping around the top of

the leg, with the thumbs pressing down on the artery. In most cases it is necessary to work underneath clothing in the groin region. Applying pressure over clothing can make the technique very difficult.

Do not apply pressure with the heel of a boot or other hard object such as a piece of wood as this can cause severe damage to the blood vessels and nerves.

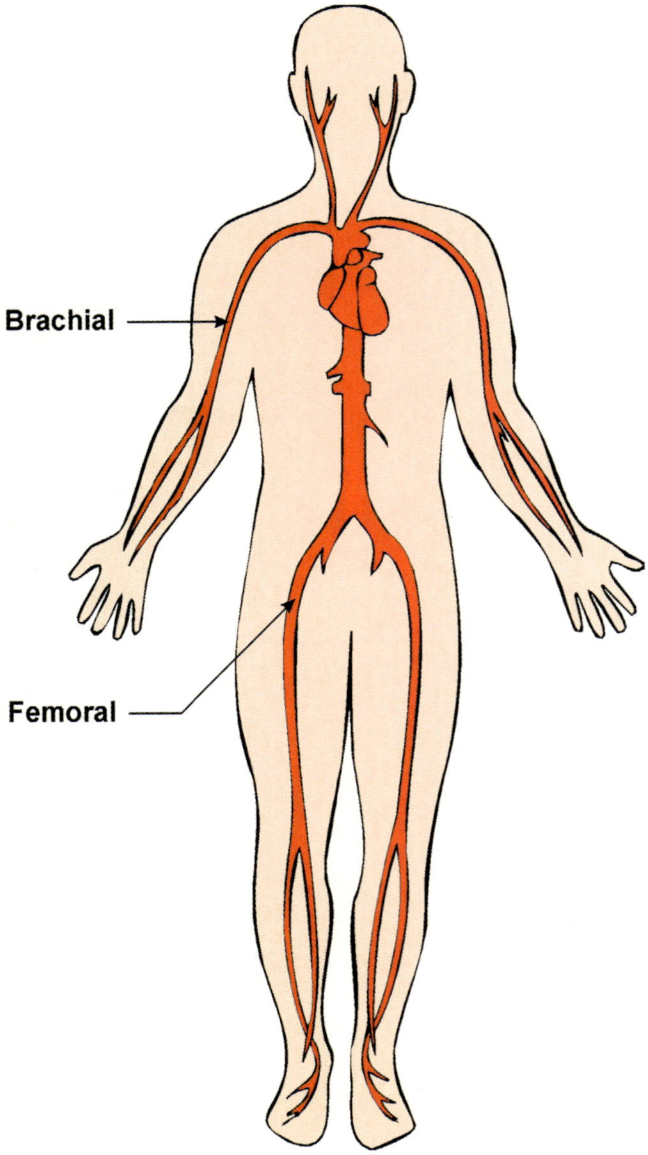

Fig.26. Pressure Points

Firm, steady pressure should be applied to a pressure point for 10 to 15 minutes. This will allow time for the clotting process to work at the site of the wound. Release of pressure should be slow, thus allowing the blood to gently flow back to the wound and minimising any disturbance of the clotting. If fresh blood begins to seep back through the third dressing, re-apply the pressure for a further 10 to 15 minutes.

Embedded Objects

In some cases there may be an embedded object in a wound, such as metal or glass. **Under no circumstances should the first aider attempt to remove the embedded object** as this can often make the problem worse by causing more damage and increasing the bleeding.

The method of application of pressure to a wound with an embedded object must be modified in such a way that the dressing does not push the object further in, yet still applies sufficient pressure to reduce or stop the bleeding.

- Place a rolled-up sterile dressing at one side of the wound. Ensure that it is placed close up to the embedded object at the edge of the wound.
- Place a second rolled-up dressing at the opposite side of the wound, again close up to the embedded object. The two rolled-up bandages should be higher than the embedded object, thus ensuring clearance for the last stage.
- Place a wound dressing over the top and secure in place. When applying pressure, do not allow the top dressing to press directly onto the embedded object.
- If the object protrudes more than a couple of inches and rises above the level of the rolled-up dressings, do not cover the protruding part. Simply secure the top dressing in place, working around the object.

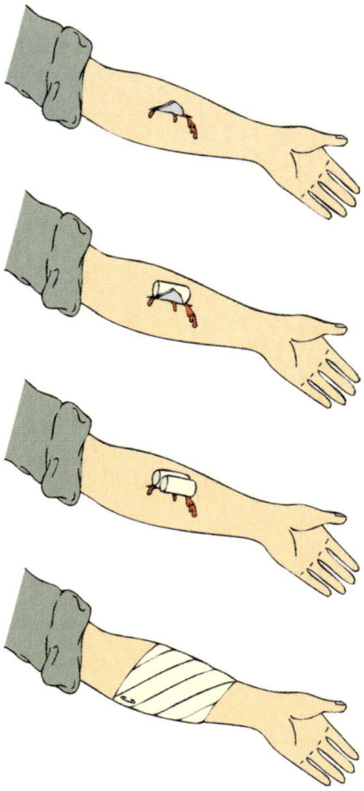

Fig.27. The Embedded Object

If an object should perforate completely through a limb, the treatment for the embedded object should be carried out at both the entry and exit points.

If the bandaging technique around a foreign or perforating object is done correctly, not only will it control the bleeding but it will also stabilise the object and stop it from moving around, preventing further damage.

Control of Bleeding from Limbs

- Put the casualty at rest. Sit or lay them down and reassure them.
- Elevate the wound above the level of the heart if possible.
- Examine the wound for any embedded object.
- Apply direct pressure to the wound with a wound dressing.
- If the wound is to an arm and the bleeding is controlled, support the arm in an elevation sling (see section 14).
- If blood seeps through the first dressing, apply a second on top of the first.
- If blood seeps through the second dressing apply a third on top of the second.
- If blood seeps through the third dressing, use indirect pressure on the nearest pressure point.

Bleeding from the Palm

The palm of the hand can be a particularly tricky part of the body to bandage, therefore a slightly different method of applying direct pressure may be needed.

If the wound is across the palm:

- Press a sterile dressing over the wound and ask the casualty to clench their fist around it. This will ensure that the wound does not gape open.
- Bandage firmly around the whole fist to maintain the pressure on the dressing.
- If the casualty is unable to clench their fist (perhaps due to broken bones to the hand or fingers), ask the casualty to hold the dressing in place and apply pressure with their uninjured hand.
- In many cases of wounds to the hand and fingers, elevation can be maintained in an elevation sling (see section 14).

If the wound is down the palm:

- Place a sterile dressing over the wound and simply bandage in place around the hand, keeping the fingers straight. If the fist is allowed to clench, it may make the wound gape open.
- Apply an elevation sling.

Amputations

If a part of the body has been amputated, treat the wound with rest, elevation, direct pressure and if necessary indirect pressure on the appropriate pressure point.

No matter how bad things may look, it is often possible for amputated parts to be re-attached, especially if they have been looked after in the correct way.

- It is important that the part is kept dry, **so do not wash it**. It should be wrapped in polythene or placed in a thin waterproof bag.
- It is also important that the part be kept cold (but not frozen), so secondly the part should be wrapped in a piece of cloth then placed in another container and surrounded by crushed ice if available.
- Mark the container containing the amputated part with the name of the casualty and the time of amputation (if known) and ensure that it is passed on to the ambulance service when they arrive.

Impalement

If a casualty is impaled on an object, do not attempt to separate them from the object as this is likely to make the injury and bleeding much worse.

- Make the casualty as comfortable as possible and, if necessary, support their body weight to relieve any tearing of the impaled part.
- Try to control any bleeding with wound dressings and, if necessary, pressure points.
- When calling for an ambulance, ensure that full details are passed on about the accident as specialist cutting tools may be needed to free the casualty.

Bleeding from the Scalp

The scalp has a very good blood supply and all wounds to the head can bleed profusely. In many cases, scalp wounds look a lot worse than they actually are but it must be remembered that with any head injury there may be some degree of damage to the brain such as concussion (see section 17).

- Make the casualty comfortable and reassure them.
- Apply a sterile dressing over the wound and bandage securely in place, applying sufficient pressure to stop the bleeding.
- Monitor the casualty for other signs and

symptoms of head injury (see section 17) and treat accordingly.

- If the bleeding is controlled and there are no signs of concussion, take the casualty to hospital for further assessment and treatment.
- If the casualty becomes unconscious, place them into the recovery position and call for an ambulance.

Bleeding from the Nose

Nose bleeds are most commonly associated with blows to the head and face although some people are prone to spontaneous nose bleeds due to no apparent reason. Blood loss occurs from very small blood vessels inside the nasal cavity.

- Sit the casualty down and lean them forward. Encourage them to spit out any blood which may be in the mouth, not to swallow it. Give the casualty a receptacle or dressing to spit the blood into.
- Advise the casualty to breathe through their mouth and pinch together the soft part of the nostrils and keep them sealed off for 10 to 15 minutes to allow time for the blood to clot.

Do not attempt to plug the nostrils.

- After 10 to 15 minutes, release the nostrils and if bleeding persists, repeat the pinching process. If bleeding still persists, take the casualty to hospital for further assessment and treatment.
- If the nose bleed was caused by direct violence, monitor the casualty for any other signs of head injury (see section 17) and treat accordingly.
- If the bleeding stops, get the casualty to clean blood from the nostrils and face and advise them to avoid exertion and not to blow their nose for a few hours as this may re-start the bleeding.

Internal Bleeding

Internal bleeding can be very difficult to diagnose as the blood loss is not visible. It usually results from direct impact or blunt trauma to the body, although it could develop as a result of certain medical conditions such as perforating ulcers. The main recognition points are:

- History of direct impact or an underlying medical condition.
- There may be pain or tenderness in the area of damage.
- Signs and symptoms of shock may be present (see section 11).

On examination, the skin above the area of damage may become discoloured. This is due to the blood seeping into the upper tissues which will eventually form a bruise.

It is virtually impossible for anyone other than a surgeon to bring internal bleeding under control but simple first aid techniques may at least reduce the bleeding and reduce the speed of deterioration.

- Lay the casualty down in a comfortable position, preferably on their back with the legs slightly raised and keep them still. If the bleeding is in the abdomen, it may be more comfortable for the casualty if the knees are drawn up to the body, thus helping to relax the abdominal muscles.
- Treat the casualty for shock (see section 11).
- If the casualty becomes unconscious, place in the recovery position and be prepared to resuscitate if necessary.
- Call for an ambulance as soon as possible.

Blood-borne Viruses

There are numerous infections which can be spread from person to person by contact with blood and other body fluids, the most well known being Hepatitis B and HIV.

Body fluids other than blood, eg vomit, saliva, sweat, tears, urine, faeces and sputum, are of very minimal risk unless containing blood. You need to take care with these, as the presence of blood is not always visible.

Blood-borne viruses are unlikely to infect a first-aider who acts hygienically. Remember, contamination with these usually occurs accidentally, for example through "sharps" (needles, broken glass). Avoid getting body fluids in open wounds, abrasions, eyes, nose or mouth, and take care if you have a skin condition like eczema.

- Always treat blood and body fluids with caution.
- Ensure that any small cuts or open wounds on your own hands are covered with adhesive dressings.
- If a wound is small and needs cleaning with fresh tap water or a moist cleansing wipe, let the casualty do this themselves.
- Wear protective gloves (latex, vinyl, polythene, etc). Be particularly careful when removing the gloves.
- Use eye protection and disposable waterproof apron if splashing is possible.
- Try as far as is practically possible to avoid contact with blood and broken skin.
- Always clean up properly after an accident. Spillages of blood will need to be disinfected (see section 1•3 and 23•1) One part bleach to ten parts cold water is a useful guide.

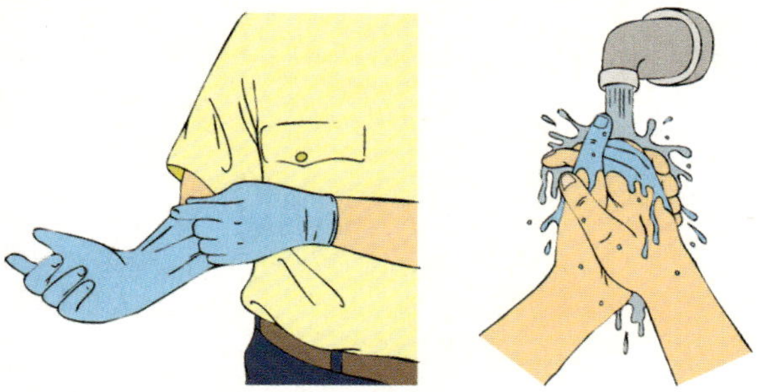

Fig.28. Basic Hygiene Measures

- When you have finished at the scene of an accident, wash your hands.

If a first-aider becomes contaminated with blood:

- wash the area with soap and water
- wash any wound with cold water and encourage it to bleed
- rinse any splashes to eyes, nose or mouth with plenty of tap water, but don't swallow it
- report it and get fast medical help - don't delay.

Test Your Knowledge

1) List 4 things you should do to protect yourself and a casualty from cross-infection, when treating an open wound:

   1 ....
   2 ....
   3 ....
   4 ....

2) Identify 4 main aims when treating someone with severe external bleeding:

   1 ....
   2 ....
   3 ....
   4 ....

3) Describe the correct positioning of casualties who are suffering from the following:

   a) Conscious - suspected angina ....
   b) Unconscious - puncture wound to right chest wall ....
   c) Unconscious - bleeding from the left ear ....
   d) Conscious - severe nose bleed ....
   e) Epilepsy - after the convulsions have ceased ....
   f) Asthma attack - ....

5) Name 3 types of bleeding from an open wound. (Place in order of severity and describe.)

   i ....

   ii ....

   iii ....

For Your Notes

Shock

Shock is a very common condition which in some cases can be life-threatening. A good knowledge and understanding of the condition is essential for all first aiders.

There are many different types of shock, each with their own individual causes and effects. First aiders in the workplace may encounter three types.

- Nervous Shock (Neurogenic)
- True Shock (Hypovolaemic)
- Allergic Shock (Anaphylactic)

Nervous Shock

This is the body's physical reaction to an overwhelming emotional stimulus.

In the early stages only reassurance is usually required but if the condition deteriorates the casualty may faint (see section 9).

In some cases, a casualty in nervous shock may begin to panic and over-react to the situation, becoming what most people would term as 'hysterical'. This panic attack may cause palpitations, trembling, sweating, crying and screaming.

Treatment

- Move the casualty to a quiet place and give lots of reassurance.
- If the casualty has a full panic attack, continue to provide reassurance but be firm and do not over-sympathise with them.
- If the casualty begins to hyperventilate, treat accordingly (see appendix G).
- Stay with the casualty until they have recovered, and advise them to consult with their doctor.

X DO NOT become aggressive, and slap the casualty's face or restrain them, as this could make them worse.

True Shock

Low (hypo) volume (vol) of blood (aemic).

This is defined as a reduction in the volume and pressure of circulating blood.

Blood exerts a certain pressure inside all blood vessels. This keeps the vessels open in their tube shape. If blood or plasma is lost from the blood vessels, the inside pressure will begin to fall and eventually the vessels may collapse. This reduces the blood and oxygen supply to the vital organs.

A reduction in blood pressure stimulating the onset of true shock can be caused by:

- blood loss;
- plasma loss from burns;
- water loss from dehydration (remember, 95% of plasma is water);
- insufficient pumping of the heart muscle, e.g. during a heart attack.

The body's reaction to a fall in blood pressure is to divert blood from less important areas of the body such as the arms, legs, skin and intestines to the most important areas in the centre of the body such as the heart muscle, brain, lung tissues and other vital organs. This natural body defence mechanism is responsible for producing most of the signs and symptoms of shock. The more the blood pressure falls, the more pronounced the signs and symptoms become.

Recognition

- The skin will become pale and feel cold to the touch, due to the warm, red blood pulling away. Cyanosis (blueness) may develop at the extremities.
- Cold skin may stimulate the casualty to shiver in an attempt to generate heat. This is not good, as the unwanted muscular activity will burn off more vital oxygen and stimulate blood flow to the limbs and main muscles, away from the vital organs.
- The casualty will begin to sweat. The nervous stimulus which controls the defence mechanism also controls the body's sweating mechanism. A cold sweat is an unwanted side effect of shock, as it means more fluid loss.
- The casualty may feel dizzy or faint. This is due to the oxygen reduction in the brain.
- The casualty may feel nauseous or may actually vomit. This feeling is often made

worse if the casualty has recently eaten or has consumed alcohol.

- The casualty may feel weak and lethargic. This is caused by a lack of oxygen and glucose (sugar) to the main muscles.
- The casualty may feel thirsty. To conserve body fluid, the salivary glands stop functioning and the mouth becomes dry. Many people have suffered this symptom as a result of dehydration, especially a hangover.
- The pulse rate will increase and gradually become weaker. To try and increase blood pressure, the heart will beat faster but as the pressure inside the arteries continues to fall, so will the amount of blood passing through them.
- The breathing rate will increase in an attempt to saturate the remaining blood with as much oxygen as possible. As it increases in speed, it becomes weak and shallow. In the later stages the casualty may begin to gasp for air.

The condition of shock is aggravated or made worse by:

- An abnormal body temperature, e.g. by becoming too warm or too cold.
- An upright posture (as gravity pulls blood into the legs, away from the vital organs).
- Eating and drinking. This may make the nausea worse and if the casualty becomes unconscious, it could contribute to vomiting.
- Smoking. Every inhalation of a cigarette puts hundreds of toxins into the blood stream which will reach the brain and other organs in just a few seconds.

Treatment

The treatment of true shock is very simple and can be very effective.

- Identify and, if possible, treat the underlying cause, e.g. control any bleeding or cool down a burn (see sections 10 and 12).
- Lay the casualty down. This stops blood pulling into the legs and increases blood flow to the brain and other vital organs.
- Elevate their legs (if injuries allow). This again helps divert blood from the legs to the vital organs.
- Maintain a normal body temperature. Wrap the casualty in a coat or blanket to help retain their natural body heat and prevent shivering.
- Keep the airway open and clear, and loosen any tight or restrictive clothing.
- Reassure the casualty throughout.
- Always call for an ambulance if a casualty should develop true shock.
- If the casualty becomes unconscious, place into the recovery position and monitor breathing and circulation.

X Do not give the casualty anything to eat or drink (including alcohol) as this may cause vomiting and may interfere with any future hospital treatments.

X Do not over-heat the casualty as this will stimulate blood flow to the extremities in an attempt to lose unwanted body heat.

X Do not allow the casualty to smoke.

Allergic Shock

This is a major allergic reaction within the body. It can be a very serious condition and, in extreme cases, life-threatening (see appendix F).

Test Your Knowledge

1) Give 4 measures you should take to treat a casualty you think is suffering from shock:

i ....

ii ....

iii ....

iv ....

2) State the effect that shock is likely to have on the following:

i Pulse ....

ii Breathing ....

iii Skin ....

iv How the casualty feels ....

Burns and Scalds

In some places of work, the risk of burns is high. Without prompt and effective first aid treatment, burns may result in severe disability, disfigurement, and possibly even a life-threatening situation.

A burn is caused by exposure to extremes of temperature, chemicals, electricity and radiation.

Burns cause two main problems.

1. **Shock**
   This is due to the loss of plasma which seeps out from the circulation and surrounding cells.
2. **Risk of Infection**
   Burned tissue offers very little resistance to invading bacteria and, if not treated correctly, the infection can become as life-threatening as the shock.

Severity of a Burn

The severity of a burn is calculated according to four factors:

- the age of the casualty
- the location of the burned area
- the depth of the burn
- the total surface area of the burn

1. **The Age of the Casualty**
   Children and elderly people are much more susceptible to the effects of burns, due to their general lack of body defence mechanisms.

2. **The Location of the Burn**
   A burn to any part of the body could be very serious, but burns to the mouth, face and neck cause even more problems. As the burned tissue begins to swell it can obstruct the airway, causing asphyxia.

3. **The Depth of a Burn**
   a. Superficial (surface).

   This is when the outermost layer of skin is burned. It causes pain, tenderness, redness and slight swelling. Small superficial burns usually heal well if prompt first aid treatment is administered. Very small superficial burns do not usually require any further medical treatment, although there may be a small risk of infection.

   b. Intermediate (partial thickness).

   This is when the burn has radiated through all the layers of skin. It causes severe pain, swelling, redness, blistering and rawness. Fluid is often visible giving the burn a shiny appearance. This is body fluid oozing from the circulation and collecting at the injured area.

   c. Deep (full thickness).

   This is when the burn has radiated down into the tissues beneath the skin. Damage is caused to nerves, fat cells, muscle and even bone. It causes intense pain, redness, swelling, deformity and distortion of the skin and in some cases the burn may become grey/black and charred. Deep burns will always require medical attention from a doctor.

4. **The Area of a Burn**
   The larger the surface area of a burn, the more fluid loss occurs and therefore the greater the degree of shock.

   A burned casualty should be sent to hospital:

   - if the casualty is a child
   - if suffering from full thickness burns
   - if suffering from burns involving the feet, hands, face or genital area
   - for all burns that extend around a limb
   - all partial thickness burns larger than 1% (the palm of the casualty's hand)
   - all superficial burns larger than 5%
   - burns of mixed depth
   - if you have any doubt about how serious the burn is.

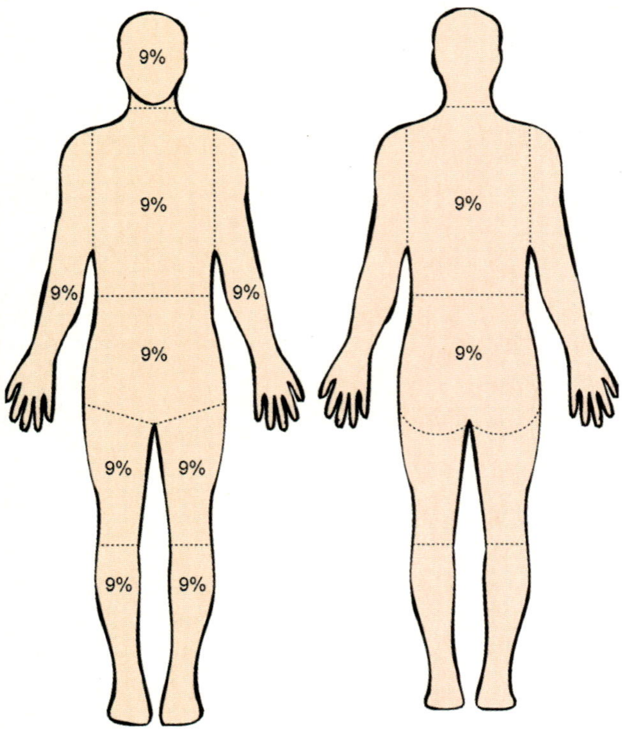

Fig.29. The Rule of Nine

As a rough guide, the surface area of the palm of the casualty's hand is worth one per cent of their total body surface. Using this as a measuring guide, the first aider should be able to calculate the approximate surface area. Burns of 9% or more will cause severe shock and the risk of infection is very high.

Burns and Scalds

The main priorities when dealing with burns are rapid cooling of the affected area and effective treatment of any developing shock.

- Ensure that the area is safe. Remember, do not become a casualty yourself.
- Ensure the source of heat is removed.
- Rest the casualty and reassure them. If the burn is severe, lay them down.
- Place the burned area under cold water for at least 10 minutes (20 minutes for chemical burns). If fresh tap water is not available, use emergency eye wash. It is good sense to ensure that a suitable water source is available in areas of the workplace where burns have been identified as a risk.
- If possible, gently remove any constricting items such as jewellery from the injured area before it begins to swell. The casualty may be able to do this themselves.
- Cover the burn with a dry, sterile wound dressing from the first aid kit.
- In the case of a minor burn, advise the casualty to watch for infection and see their doctor if it becomes evident. If ever in doubt about the severity of even a small burn, seek further medical aid from a doctor or hospital.
- In the case of a severe burn, call for an ambulance and keep cooling the burn until it arrives. The ambulance crew will cover the burn, perhaps with specialised dressings.
- Treat the casualty for shock (see section 11) and monitor for deterioration.
- If the casualty becomes unconscious, place them in the recovery position but remember to keep cooling the burn. The effects of a burn do not disappear just because a casualty has become unconscious.

Things to Avoid in the Treatment of Burns and Scalds

- DO NOT apply any fat, cream, lotions or oil based substances to the burn as this can increase the burning effect and interfere with the natural healing process.
- DO NOT remove any clothing which is stuck to the burned area as this may peel off the skin and cause more damage. Simply pour the water over the whole area.
- DO NOT break any blisters which may have formed around the burn. This would result in more fluid loss and allow infection below the skin.
- DO NOT put adhesive dressings or tape onto the burned area.

Burns to the Airway

These can be caused by hot or corrosive liquids or the inhalation of very hot air, e.g. from an explosion. As well as shock and infection, burns around the neck and face and inside the mouth and air passages have the associated problem of swelling, causing airway obstruction and asphyxia.

The main aim of treatment is to cool the burned tissue if possible, and to maintain an adequate and open airway.

- If the burn is to the outside of the neck or face, cool it with wet cloths and keep them wet.
- If the burn is to the inside of the mouth and throat, give the casualty ice to suck or cold water to rinse out the mouth. DO NOT put anything inside the mouth if you think that the casualty may choke. If ice is given, break it up into small pieces. DO NOT let the casualty swallow the ice or water as this will cool the body and increase the shock.
- Put the casualty in a position which best helps breathing and loosen any tight or restrictive clothing.

- If the burn is severe, or any airway or breathing problems develop, call for an ambulance.
- Monitor the level of consciousness and breathing. If unconscious, place the casualty into the recovery position. If breathing stops, carry out resuscitation.

Chemical Burns

Certain chemicals (acid and alkali) can burn and absorb into the body tissue.

- Ensure the safety of yourself and the casualty. Do not become contaminated yourself by the chemical (remember, liquids can also give off gases and fumes). If appropriate, wear protective clothing.
- Flood the affected area with copious amounts of water. This will not only cool the burn but will also dilute and disperse the chemical. When doing this, be careful not to splash or swill the chemical to unaffected areas.
- Keep cooling the burn for at least 20 minutes or until an ambulance arrives.
- If the burn is minor, cover it with a dry, sterile dressing and seek further medical aid. If the chemical has absorbed into the body tissue it can continue to burn for many hours, therefore all chemical burns should be seen by a doctor as soon as possible.
- If the burn is severe, treat for shock as appropriate and monitor the level of consciousness and breathing.
- In all cases of chemical burns and contamination, pass on details of the chemical to the doctor or hospital.

Electrical Burns

Caused by a lightning strike or by low or high voltage current, electrical burns can develop all over the body, even though the point of entry may be quite specific.

Deep (full thickness) burns usually occur at the point of contact, but as the current radiates to all parts of the body, superficial and intermediate burns can develop internally and externally.

As a secondary effect, the current can cause serious damage to the normal electrical signals in the body, resulting in unconsciousness, respiratory and circulatory arrest.

- If appropriate, and if possible, disconnect the electricity supply to ensure the safety of yourself and the casualty. If you cannot disconnect the electricity supply, call for specialist assistance. Remember, do not become a casualty yourself.
- Resuscitate the casualty if necessary.
- Cool any obvious burns (especially the contact area) with water for at least 10 minutes. If the casualty is unconscious, they will not be able to indicate the areas of pain so examine for signs of burns all over the body.
- Once cooled, cover the burn with a dry sterile dressing.
- Even in cases of minor electrical burns, the casualty must seek immediate medical attention from a doctor or hospital.
- If the casualty is unconscious, place them in the recovery position and monitor breathing and circulation.

X It may seem obvious, but in the panic DO NOT let the water and electricity come together.

Test Your Knowledge

1) A colleague has spilt hot tea on her foot. You should immediately (please tick one answer):

a) lay her flat, with foot raised   b) immerse her foot in a bowl of cold water
c) put burn spray all over area   d) cover with a dressing and take to hospital

2) A casualty with throat burns is *most* in danger from (please tick one answer):

a) infection   b) fainting
c) breathing difficulties   d) internal damage

3) Three things you *should not* do when treating a burn are:

i .... ii .... iii ....

Injuries to Muscles & Joints

Although not usually life-threatening, injuries to joints and the soft tissue which surrounds them can sometimes be very serious.

The skeleton is a very articulate structure which allows movement in many different places due to the large number of movable joints.

The muscles of the body have many functions but their main function is to provide movement to the skeletal framework. Muscles are connected to bones by tendons. The ligaments of the body join bone to bone across joints, only allowing the joint a certain amount or range of movement.

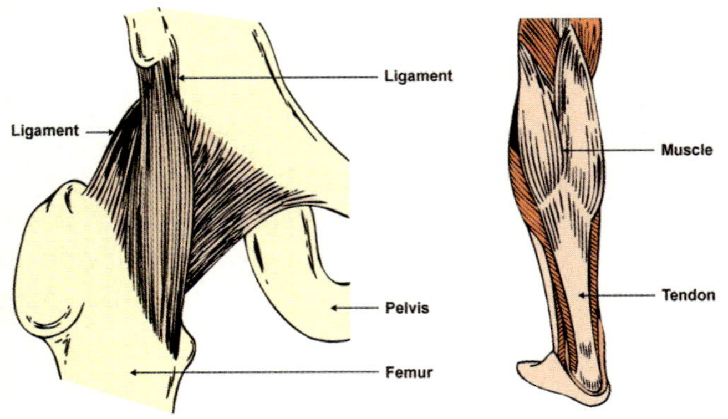

Fig.30 Muscles, Tendons and Ligaments

In general, muscles, tendons and ligaments are robust structures, capable of taking impact and trauma in their stride but in some cases they are subject to overwhelming force, causing damage.

Muscular Strains

A muscular strain occurs when muscles are over-stretched or twisted into abnormal positions, causing them to tear.

Muscular strains are the commonest single cause of absenteeism from work every year in the UK, the main cause for injury being attributed to the incorrect manual handling and movement of loads.

Recognition points of a muscular strain may include:

- history of physical activity or stretching.
- localised pain which is made worse on movement.
- weakness and partial loss of function in the area of pain.
- in severe cases, possible swelling and bruising at the site of pain.

Sprains

A sprain occurs when a joint is forced past its normal range of movement.

This causes damage to muscle and tendons but in particular to the ligaments around the joint which are over-stretched.

Recognition points of a sprain may include:

- history of twisting or wrenching the joint.
- pain and tenderness. In some cases the pain can be intense, resembling that of a fracture.
- swelling and possible bruising around the joint.
- loss of power and function at the joint.

Treatment of strains and sprains

First aid treatment of muscular strains and sprains is very basic and revolves around the need to prevent the injury from worsening.

- **R** - Rest the casualty, in particular the injured area.
- **I** - Immobilise the area if possible. For example, if the injury is to a shoulder, place the arm into an elevation sling (see section 14).
- **C** - Cold Compress. If ice is not available in the workplace, a simple wet dressing held on the area for approximately 20 minutes will help reduce swelling and pain. If ice is used, it should wrapped in a cloth and not allowed to come into direct contact with the skin.
- **E** - Elevate the area if possible to help reduce swelling.
- If work is likely to make the injury worse, the casualty should be sent to see a doctor at the earliest possible opportunity. If they carry on working with an already damaged muscle or joint, the injury is likely to worsen.
- In the case of minor muscular strains, advise the casualty to see their doctor if the condition worsens or becomes persistent.
- In all cases of sprains it is best to be on the safe side. Therefore, the casualty should be sent or taken to hospital for further examination. You never know, there may be a fracture to the underlying bone.

X The application of heat to the injured area to stimulate blood flow and healing is not classified as a first aid measure (it's a physiotherapy practice) therefore heat packs, sprays and creams should not be used unless advised by the company nurse or the casualty's doctor.

Dislocations

A dislocation is the displacement of a bone from its natural position.

In some cases, when the bones have automatically gone back into place, it may look very much like a severe sprain although the pain is usually much worse. In other cases, the bones may remain out of their normal position in which case the deformity can be extreme.

Recognition points of a dislocation may include:

- history of violence or wrenching to the injured joint.
- intense pain and tenderness. The pain can be so severe that it may radiate to other areas.
- swelling, bruising and deformity of the joint.
- loss of function and power to the affected part.
- dislocations to the larger joints such as the knee, hip, elbow and shoulder may cause severe complications such as damage to organs, nerves and blood vessels. This may result in severe shock which is further aggravated by the pain.

All dislocations are very serious injuries and will require some form of further medical treatment at a hospital. First aid treatment is simply designed to prevent the injury worsening.

Treatment

- Immobilise the injured area as for a fracture (see section 14) to prevent further movement of the bones and joint. In most cases, it is best to immobilise in the position found.
- If the dislocation is to the wrist or finger(s), keep the injured part elevated if possible.
- If appropriate, call for an ambulance to ensure comfortable transportation to hospital.
- If appropriate, treat for shock.

X NEVER try to replace or 'reduce' a dislocation. This can cause immense damage to soft tissue, blood vessels and nerves.

Test Your Knowledge

1) Describe:

a) A sprain ....

b) A strain ....

c) A dislocation ....

2) The treatment for a sprain is:

r......................... i......................... c......................... e.........................

Fractures

Fractures can be very serious injuries, and although not usually life-threatening, poor management at the scene of the accident can result in more damage and long term disability.

The skeleton is made up of many bones of different shapes and sizes. Bone tissue is mainly comprised of calcium which gives toughness and strength, although the honeycombed arrangement of inner bone structure reduces weight.

A fracture is defined as a crack, chip or break in the continuity of a bone.

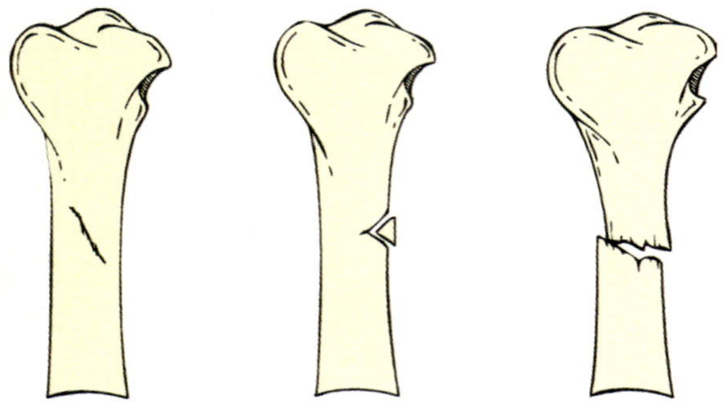

Fig. 31. Definitions of a Fracture

Types of Fracture

1. Closed (Simple) Fracture

This is when the bone is fractured but there is no associated open wound, although bruising may be evident. In cases of cracks and chips, simple fractures can be difficult to diagnose without the aid of x-rays.

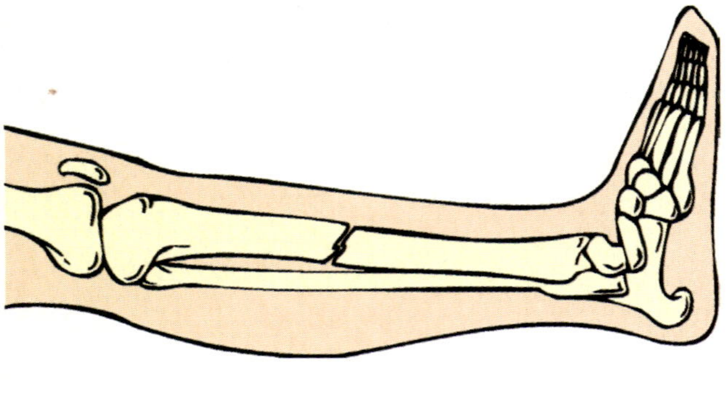

Fig.32. Closed (Simple) Fracture

2. Open (Compound) Fracture

This is when the bone is fractured and there is also an associated open wound. In some cases the broken bone ends may protrude through the wound. The control of bleeding and prevention of further infection into the broken bone ends are major considerations in the treatment.

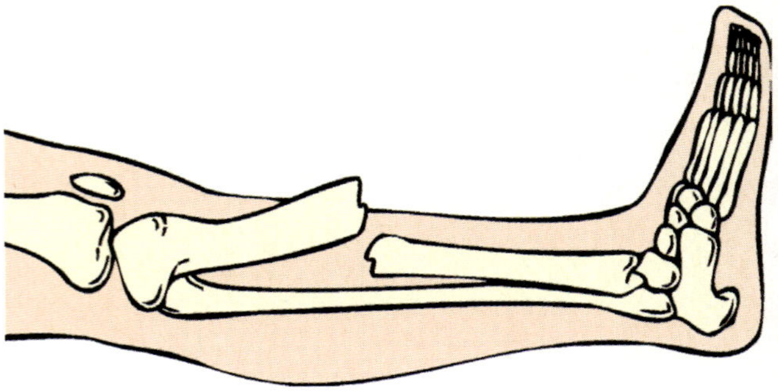

Fig.33. Open (Compound) Fracture

3. Complicated Fracture

This is when the fracture causes damage to, or interference with, organs or other important structures. Examples are broken ribs causing lung damage, or a broken forearm causing damage to blood vessels. The commonest type of complication is when broken bone ends trap blood vessels and restrict circulation which can have very serious consequences. Both open and closed fractures can be complicated.

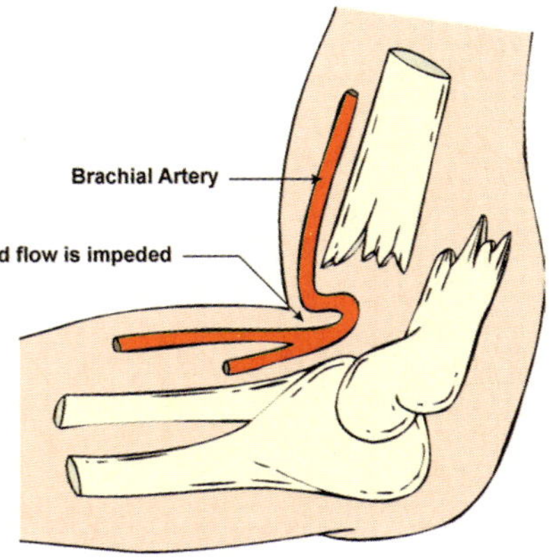

Fig.34. Complicated Fracture

Causes of Fractures

1. Direct Force

This is the most common cause of a fracture, when the bone fractures at the point of impact.

2. Indirect Force

This is when the bone fractures away from the point of impact. As bone is solid, it will transmit shock waves along its length.

Examples of this are:

- a fall onto the outstretched arm. The point of impact is the heel of the hand but the shock wave travels up the braced arm to the weak point in the shoulder causing a fracture to the collar bone (clavicle);
- a fall onto the heels of the feet. The points of impact are the heels but the shock wave travels up the braced leg, through the pelvis and up the spine. Weak points exist at the hip, all the way up the spine and the base of the skull.

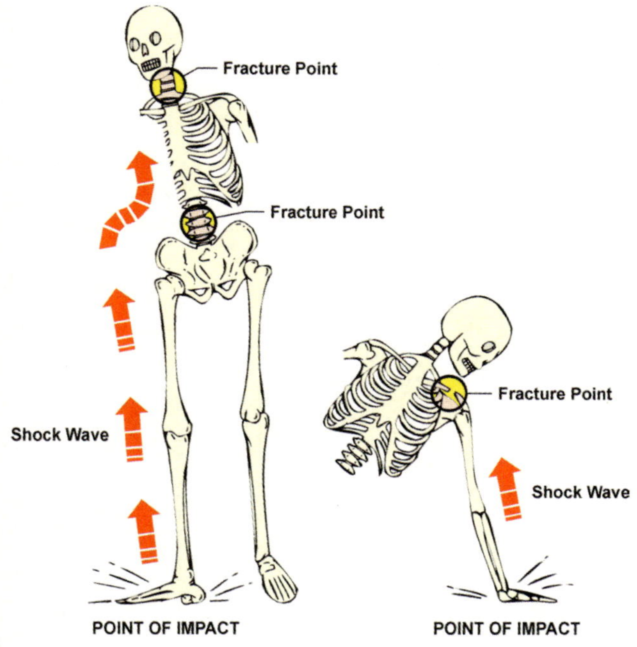

Fig.35. Indirect Force

3. Muscular Action

Many muscles are responsible for providing movement to the skeleton. In some cases, the force created by contracting muscles can be sufficient to fracture bone to which they are attached.

Fractures to Upper Limbs

The recognition points of a fracture to a bone of the upper limb may vary considerably, dependent on the type of fracture and the size of the bone involved. The following is a basic guide.

Recognition

Bones of the Upper Limb
Fingers (Phalanges)
Hand (Metacarpals)
Wrist (Carpals)
Forearm (Radius and Ulna)
Upper Arm (Humerus)
Shoulder and Collar bone (Scapula and Clavicle)

- History of impact, or violence to the area.
- Pain and tenderness.
- Bruising and swelling. This can be extensive if large blood vessels have been damaged.
- Deformity. This can be extensive if long bones have broken clean through.
- Loss of power and function.
- Crepitus may be heard (this is the sound made by broken bone ends as they rub together). This should never be purposely tested for!
- Shock.

Treatment

The general rules in the management of all upper limb fractures are:

- if the fracture is open, control any bleeding as the priority. If bone ends protrude from the wound, bandage in the same way as for embedded objects (see section 10). Ensure that any protruding bone ends are gently covered with a sterile dressing to prevent infection getting into the bone;
- stop the injury worsening by providing support and immobilisation. If broken bones are allowed to move, it will cause more pain and may cause further damage to blood vessels and other soft tissue at the fracture site;
- support and immobilise the injured part in a comfortable position. The exact position for immobilisation and support will be dependent on the comfort of the casualty. If the chosen position for immobilisation increases the pain and discomfort, it would indicate that it is probably making the condition worse. DO NOT attempt to move the injured part unnecessarily or force it into an uncomfortable position.

An ideal way of providing comfortable and effective support and immobilisation for an upper limb is with the use of a sling.

There are two main types of sling used in first aid, the elevation sling and the arm sling. To apply a sling, you will need a triangular bandage from the first aid kit.

- **The Elevation Sling**

  This sling is ideal for immobilising injuries to the fingers, wrist or hand as it keeps the injured part in an elevated position which helps reduce swelling and further discomfort.

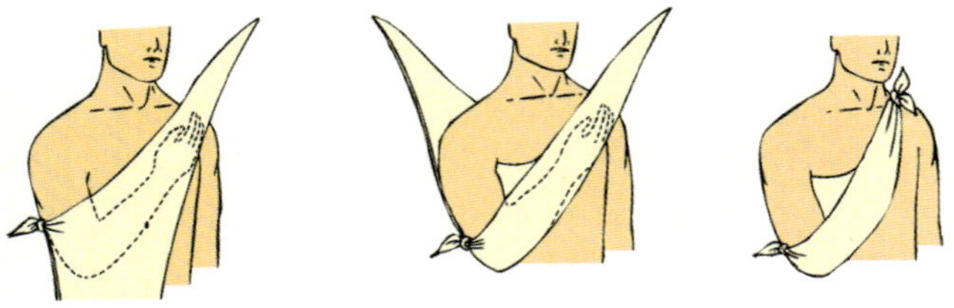

Fig.36. The Elevation Sling

- **The Arm Sling**

  This sling supports the arm in a position at right angles across the body. It is ideal for injuries to the upper arm and forearm.

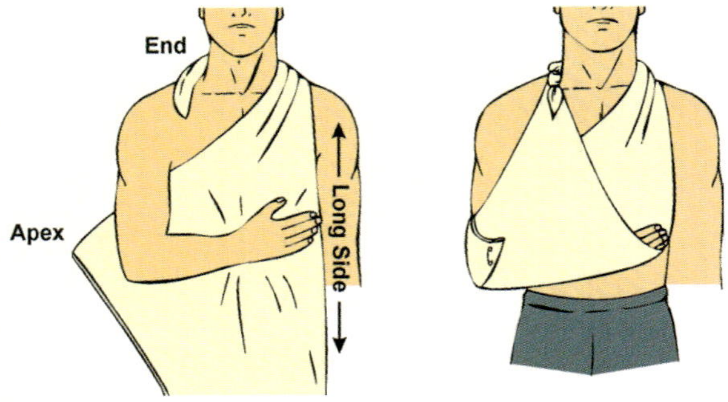

Fig.37. The Arm Sling

- always check for circulation in the limb. Circulation may be restricted by swelling or perhaps rings or a watch. If circulation is restricted, it may make the affected part go cold, change colour (usually pale) and the casualty may complain of numbness or a tingling sensation;
- if the fracture is severe, do not attempt to transport the casualty to hospital, as walking and moving may aggravate the problem. Call for an ambulance;
- always watch for shock. In some cases this may be severe.

The following paragraphs indicate simple methods of treatment when dealing with fractures of bones to the upper limbs, although it must be appreciated that there are many similar but different ways of achieving the same results.

1. Fractures of the Fingers and Hand

In most cases, the fingers will adopt a slightly curved, 'cupped' shape. This is usually the most comfortable position for immobilisation.

- Rest the casualty and reassure them.
- Look for any circulation restriction caused by jewellery. If present, ask the casualty to carefully remove the jewellery. If removal is not possible or causes any further pain or discomfort, leave it in place but ensure that the casualty is taken to hospital quickly and the hospital are informed of the circulation problem.
- Place a ball of soft padding in the cup of the hand. This will stop the fingers moving inward.
- Gently but firmly wrap a broad bandage around the outside of the hand. This will stop the fingers moving outward. This should not be so tight as to cause further pain to the casualty
- Apply an elevation sling to help reduce swelling.
- Take the casualty to hospital for further treatment.

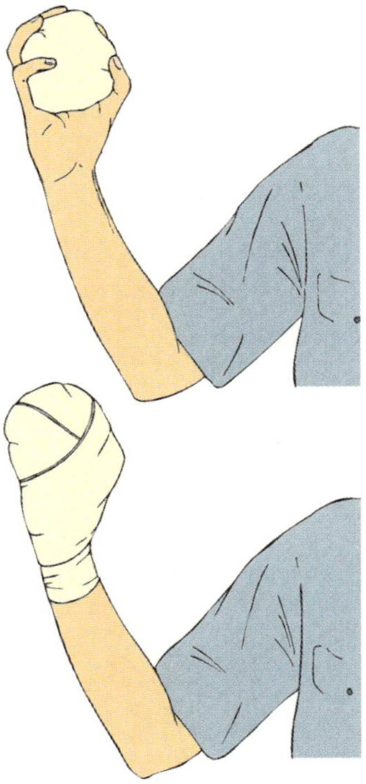

Fig.38. Fractured Hand and Fingers

2. Fractures of the Wrist

The main aim is to stop the wrist joint from moving and reduce swelling.

- Rest the casualty and reassure them.
- Gently pad around the wrist with soft material.
- Keep the wrist rested by applying an arm sling. Secure a broad bandage around the body, overlapping the elbow of the injured arm. This will stop the arm moving by using the body as a splint.
- Monitor circulation in the hand.

- Take the casualty to hospital or, if in doubt, call for an ambulance.

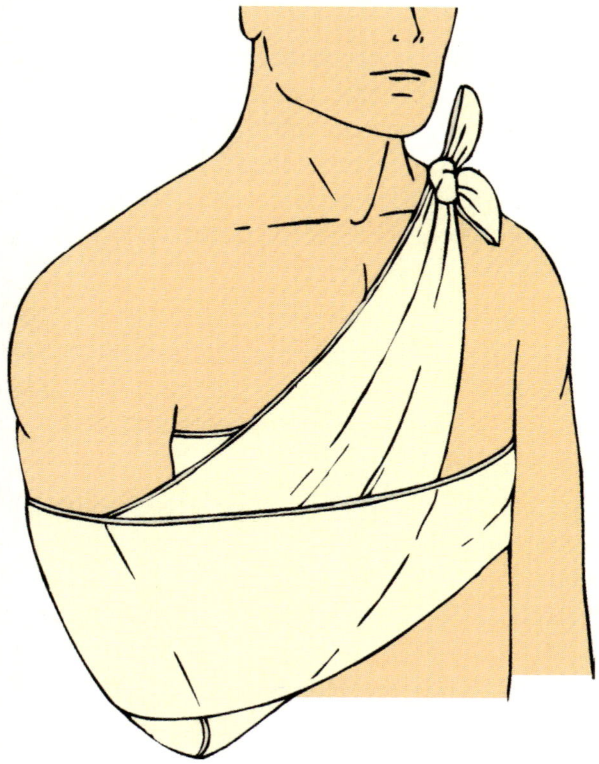

Fig.39. Fractured Hand and Fingers

3. Fractures of the Forearm and Upper Arm

These can be very serious injuries. The forearm and upper arm bones are long; therefore, if they are broken clean through it will form a long, sharp-ended lever which can cause damage to soft tissue, nerves and large blood vessels. Fractures to the long bones of the arm should ideally be transported to hospital by ambulance.

The main aim of treatment is to provide immobilisation and support to the fracture site so the broken bone ends cannot move independently of each other.

- If the casualty can move the arm without causing discomfort and the fracture is only suspected to be a crack or chip to the bone, the arm should be placed in a sling (with a broad bandage around the body to provide further immobilisation, for the forearm).
- If the bone is broken clean through, gently place soft sterile dressings around the fracture site and, if possible, try to support the arm in the position in which it was found. If possible, use the most appropriate sling (and secure the arm to the body with a broad bandage, for the forearm).

  If the arm is found in such a position that it will not go into a sling, e.g it is straight, simply pad around the fracture site to immobilise it and call for an ambulance.
- Check circulation in the hand. If circulation is not present, do nothing, but ensure that this information is passed on when calling for the ambulance.
- Monitor for shock and treat as appropriate.

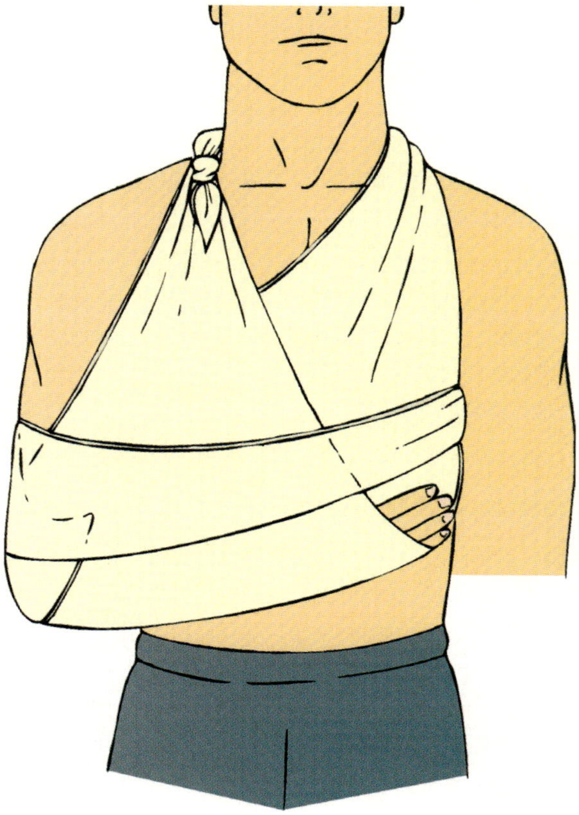

Fig.40. Fractures to the Lower Arm and Wrist

4. Fractures around the Elbow Joint

This can be a very serious injury as the broken bone ends can cause damage to the main blood vessels and nerve pathways which pass across the joint.

X DO NOT attempt to bend or move the joint at all.

- Immobilise the arm in the position found, using a sling if appropriate.
- Monitor for shock and treat as appropriate.
- Check circulation at the wrist by feeling for the radial pulse. If circulation is not present, do nothing, but ensure that this information is passed on when calling for the ambulance.

5. Fractures of the Collar Bone

This is a very common fracture, the main cause of which is indirect force. The collar bone usually runs very close to the surface of the skin and a clean break can cause obvious deformity, usually in the form of a raised lump or ridge.

Although not a true bone of the arm, if the arm on the injured side is allowed to move it will put pressure onto the broken collar bone and cause more damage and pain. The main aim of treatment is to immobilise the arm on the injured side.

- Rest the casualty and reassure them.

- If possible, support the arm in an elevation sling and pad the natural hollow between the body and the elbow. Place a broad bandage around the elbow and secure to the body (as for a fractured wrist).

  If it is not possible to move the arm into the elevated position, support the arm at right angles to the body in an arm sling and secure the arm to the body with a broad bandage.

- When secured in position, check for circulation in the arm by feeling for the radial pulse. If circulation is not present, do nothing, but ensure that this information is passed on when calling for the ambulance.
- Monitor for shock and treat as appropriate.

6. Fractures of the Shoulder Blade

The shoulder blade (scapula) is a large flat bone and fractures to it are not common due to the high amount of impact needed. Although not a true bone of the arm, if the arm on the injured side is allowed to move it will cause movement of the fracture site.

Treatment is the same as for the collar bone.

Fractures to Lower Limbs

The recognition points of a fracture to a bone of the lower limb may vary considerably, dependent on the type of fracture and the size of the bone involved. The following is a basic guide.

Recognition

Bones of the Lower Limb
Toes (Phalanges)
Foot (Metatarsals)
Ankle (Tarsals)
Lower Leg (Tibia and Fibula)
Upper Leg (Femur)

- History of impact, or violence to the area.
- Pain and tenderness.
- Bruising and swelling. This can be extensive if large blood vessels have been damaged.
- Deformity. This can be extensive if long bones have broken clean through.
- Loss of power and function.
- Crepitus may be heard (this is the sound made by broken bone ends as they rub together). This should never be purposely tested for!
- Shock. A casualty can lose over three pints of blood internally with a fractured femur.

Treatment

The general rules in the management of all lower limb fractures are:

- if the fracture is open, control any bleeding as the priority. If bone ends protrude from the wound, bandage in the same way as for embedded objects (see section 10). Ensure that any protruding bone ends are gently covered with a sterile dressing to prevent infection getting into the bone;
- stop the injury worsening by providing support and immobilisation. If broken bones are allowed to move, it will cause more pain and may cause further damage to blood vessels and other soft tissue at the fracture site;
- support and immobilise the injured part in a comfortable position. The exact position for immobilisation and support will be dependent on the comfort of the casualty. DO NOT attempt to move the injured part unnecessarily or force it into an uncomfortable position;
- always check for circulation in the limb. Swelling and deformity are the main causes of circulation restriction in a fractured leg. If circulation is restricted, it may make the affected part go cold, change colour (usually pale) and the casualty may complain of numbness or a tingling sensation;
- if the fracture is to the long bones of the upper and lower leg or the knee cap, do not attempt to transport the casualty to hospital, as walking and moving will aggravate the problem. Call for an ambulance;
- always watch for shock. In some cases this may be severe.

The following paragraphs indicate simple methods of treatment when dealing with fractures of bones to the lower limbs, although it must be appreciated that there are many similar but different ways of achieving the same results.

1. Fractures of the Toes and Foot

These are mainly caused by crushing under a heavy object.

- Rest the casualty and do not let them walk on the injured foot.
- Ask the casualty if they can remove their shoe or boot from the injured foot. However, if this causes more pain, or swelling is so great that the footwear will not come off, leave it in place.
- Keep the injured part elevated to reduce swelling and, if possible, apply a cold compress to the injured area.

- Arrange for the casualty to be taken to hospital, maintaining elevation of the foot if possible.

2. Fractures of the Ankle, Lower and Upper Leg

These can be very serious injuries and should always be fully immobilised with splints before transportation to hospital. In the majority of circumstances, first aiders in the workplace will not have access to purpose made splints so an ambulance will be needed.

- Rest and reassure the casualty and support their body in the most comfortable position.
- Provide support and immobilisation to the injured area with soft padding.
- Monitor the casualty for shock and treat accordingly. However, do not attempt to elevate the injured leg if this is likely to make the condition worse.
- Call for an ambulance.

3. Fractures around the Knee Joint and Knee Cap

These are treated in the same way as fractures to the lower leg (above), although it must be stressed that any movement of the joint, in any direction, must be avoided. This could cause serious damage to large blood vessels and nerve pathways which pass across the joint.

Splinting a Fractured Leg

If the first aider is responsible for the transportation of the casualty to hospital, or if the accident has happened in a remote area where the ambulance is likely to take a long time to arrive, it may be beneficial to straighten and splint the injured leg.

If the first aider is expected to use a purpose-made splint as a part of their first aid duties, they should receive specific and specialised instruction on how to use it.

If specialised equipment is not available, it is often possible to improvise by using the uninjured leg as a splint.

- Support the casualty in a comfortable position and reassure them. Tell them what you are about to do.
- Gently and carefully straighten the injured leg in line with the uninjured leg. Do this slowly and advise the casualty to take deep breaths and to try to relax. Provide maximum support to the leg and injury site when straightening the leg.
- Place soft padding in any natural hollows between the two legs.
- If the injury is to the ankle, secure the feet together by placing broad bandages around the toes and shins. Do not tie a bandage directly over the site of injury.
- If the injury is not to the ankle, secure the feet and ankles together with a 'figure of eight' bandage. For this you will need a broad bandage.

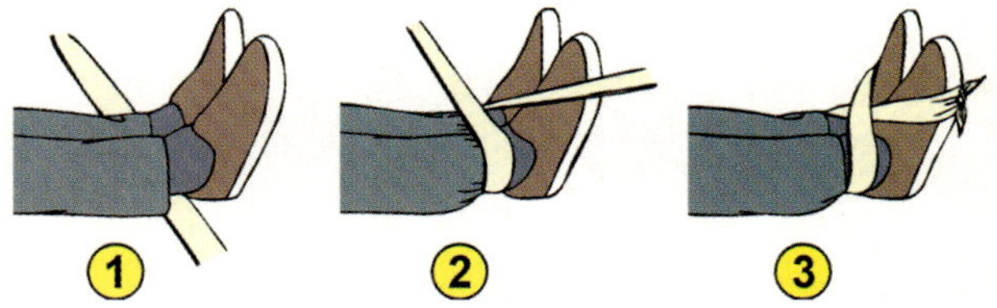

Fig.41. Figure of Eight Bandage

- Gently slide more broad bandages under the ankles and knees. Fold them around the two legs and tie them off on the uninjured side. Use more broad bandages if necessary to secure the two legs together but do not place one directly over the site of injury.

Fractures to The Pelvis and Hip

Fractures to the pelvis are a very serious injury and in many cases can be life-threatening due to internal bleeding. Fractures to the pelvis can also cause damage to internal organs such as the bladder.

Recognition

The Pelvis and Hip
• History of impact, or violence to the area.
• Pain and tenderness in the hip, groin or lower back which is made worse if the casualty moves.
• Inability to stand or move the legs, even though the legs are uninjured.
• The casualty may feel the sensation of wanting to pass water.
• Shock.

Treatment

Treatment of a fractured pelvis or hip bone is exactly the same as for fractures to the upper leg, but in addition:

- if the casualty feels the need to pass water, discourage them from doing so as this may cause more complications such as infection.
- if the casualty is lying on their back, it may make the casualty more comfortable if the knees are bent slightly and supported underneath.

Back Injuries and Suspected Spinal Fractures

For many first aiders, spinal injuries are one of the most daunting types of injury to have to deal with. It is quite correct to have a good appreciation as to how severe the injury could be, but a first aider should at all times remain focused on the priorities of airway, breathing and circulation and carry out any necessary treatments with confidence and attention to detail.

The spinal cord passes down through the centre of the spinal column which is made up of bones called vertebrae. It carries messages between the brain and most parts of the body, and if it is damaged, the effects can be widespread.

There are many possible types of back injury, ranging from a simple pulled muscle to a compressed or severed spinal cord. In some cases, determining the exact nature and extent of the injury can be very difficult for the first aider, so the golden rule is to always suspect the worst possible injury and to treat accordingly.

Recognition

The Spine
● History of impact, violence or twisting of the back or neck. "Read the accident". ● There may be some form of deformity in the continuity of the spine. ● Possible pain and tenderness at the site of injury, although this pain may be masked by other injuries. ● There may be a total or partial loss of power, function and feeling in the arms or legs. ● The casualty may feel tingling sensations in the limbs. ● Shock. Spinal injuries often make the blood pressure fall.

Treatment

- Do not move the casualty unless it is absolutely necessary, e.g. due to an uncontrollable danger.
- Keep the casualty still and reassure them.
- If a bystander or helper is available, get them to gently hold and support the casualty's head in the jaw thrust position. If there is a bystander available, use a rolled up coat or other firm padding to stop the head moving.
- If the casualty is conscious, pad all around the casualty with coats etc., ensuring that the whole body is fully supported and immobilised in the position found.
- Cover the casualty with a coat or blanket to help maintain body temperature.
- Call for an ambulance and ensure that details relating to the cause and severity of the injury are passed on, but be discreet, do not alarm the casualty with worrying comments.
- If vomiting, or unconscious and you need to leave the casualty, use a recovery position (see section 9.6).

Fractures to the Skull, Jaw and Face

There are many individual bones which make up the skull and face and the usual cause of fracture is direct impact.

Recognition

The Skull, Jaw and Face
● History of impact, or violence to the head. ● Pain and tenderness at the site of injury. ● There may be deformity such as a lump or indentation at the site of injury. ● Bruising and swelling. ● Signs and symptoms of concussion or compression may be evident (see section 17). ● The casualty may bleed from the nose or wound to the skin.

Treatment

- In all cases:
    - ensure the casualty's mouth is clear of any saliva, blood or broken teeth;
    - if the casualty is unconscious, place them into the recovery position and monitor breathing;
    - control any obvious bleeding;
    - monitor for any signs of concussion or compression injury to the brain and treat accordingly (see section 17);
    - reassure the casualty at all times and keep them at rest;
    - seek further medical aid in the most appropriate way.
- For the jaw bone:
    - if conscious, lean the casualty forward slightly and encourage them to spit out any saliva or blood onto a dressing pad rather than swallow it. Swallowing will cause movement of the jaw which is likely to increase pain;

- get the casualty to support their jaw with soft padding.

- For the facial bones, e.g. cheek and nose:
  - apply a cold compress to the area to reduce swelling and bruising and to ease the pain.
- For the skull:
  - if fluid is leaking from the ear, cover the ear with a sterile dressing to prevent infection getting into the skull and treat as for compression injury (see section 17). If the casualty has to be placed into the recovery position, place them with the leaking ear lowermost to allow drainage and reduce the build up of pressure inside the skull.

Fractures to the Ribcage

See Chest Injuries (section 15)

Crush Injuries

These are caused when a part of the body is trapped or crushed under a heavy object. Injury can be extensive, with bleeding, shock and fractures present.

If a limb has been crushed for even a short period of time, there are two serious complications which could develop. Shock and crush syndrome.

1. Extensive shock, especially when the crushing object is removed from the limb and fluid leaks from surrounding tissue into the damaged area.
2. Crush Syndrome. This occurs when damaged tissues release toxic substances into the trapped circulation. These toxins build up to such a high level that if released suddenly into the general circulation, they can cause kidney failure and death.

- In all cases of crush injuries:
  - monitor the casualty for shock and treat as appropriate (see section 11);
  - when calling for an ambulance, pass on information relating to the nature of the crushing object and the duration of the crush. Specialist rescue equipment and medical skills may be necessary at the scene. The ambulance service must always be informed that it is a crush injury, even if the trapped limb has already been released.
- If the limb has been crushed for less than 15 minutes:
  - if possible, and if enough helpers are available to make it safe, release the limb as a matter of urgency;
  - control any bleeding and immobilise and support any fractures.
- If the limb has been crushed for more than 15 minutes:

X DO NOT release the limb;

  - control any bleeding as best you can, using indirect pressure on the pressure points if necessary;
  - support the casualty in the most comfortable position possible, using padding if available.

Test Your Knowledge

1) You are called to deal with a casualty who is trapped by a heavy crate across his legs. He is conscious and can answer your questions. He is in a great deal of pain and you note that the skin of the legs is cool and blue.
   a) What must you find out before releasing the crate? ....
   b) When would it be safe to release the casualty? ....
   c) What could happen to the casualty if treated incorrectly, and why?..........
   ....

3) Describe:
   a) A closed fracture ....
   b) An open fracture ....
   c) A complicated fracture ....

4) What are some of the dangers of a fractured jaw? a)..........
   b) ....

5) Spinal fractures are serious because of possible injury to the..........

Chest Injuries

Although not common, all chest injuries have the potential of becoming very serious, causing both asphyxia and shock.

The chest wall is made up of twelve pairs of ribs which connect to the breastbone at the front and to the spine at the back. In general, the chest wall is a robust structure which provides a good amount of protection to the important organs inside the chest cavity.

Injuries to the chest include fractured ribs, penetrating wounds and internal bleeding, all of which could quite easily be life-threatening.

The usual cause of chest injuries is direct impact, resulting from a fall or a blow to the chest. Some places and types of work may have specific hazards which can result in chest injury: for example, police officers, security guards and military personnel. These people often wear protective vests or jackets due to the increased risk.

Fractured Ribs

In many cases, the injury is simply a small crack to one or two of the ribs which, although painful, does not usually cause any serious breathing problems for the casualty. In some cases, however, there may be multiple fractures of the ribs, which is very serious.

Recognition

With a single fractured rib there may be:

- history of impact or a blow to the chest wall;
- pain and tenderness at the site of injury;
- the injured area may be bruised and slightly swollen;
- shallow breathing. The pain is often made worse if the casualty takes deep breaths;
- a slight reduction in the movement of the arm on the injured side. The pain is often made worse if this arm is allowed to move, as it stretches the muscles between the ribs.

With multiple broken ribs there may be:

- history of impact or a blow to the chest wall;
- severe pain and tenderness at the site of injury which is made worse if the casualty takes a deep breath;
- the chest wall may be bruised and there may be obvious deformity;
- a portion of the chest wall may lose its rigidity due to the multiple fractures (flail), causing the chest wall to move inward when the casualty inhales. This movement of the chest wall in the opposite direction to normal (paradoxical movement) is caused by the vacuum inside the chest, sucking the fractured ribs inward;
- breathing will be shallow and distressed;
- pale, clammy skin and blueness may be present at the extremities;
- the casualty may cough up blood which may be bright red and frothy. This indicates internal damage to the lung.

Treatment

For a single fractured rib:

- rest and reassure the casualty;
- support the arm on the injured side in an elevation sling to reduce movement of the chest muscles;
- take the casualty to hospital for further examination and treatment;
- if at any time the casualty begins to develop serious breathing difficulties, shock, or coughing up blood, treat as for multiple broken ribs (below).

For multiple broken ribs:

- rest the casualty in the position which best helps their breathing. This is often laid down with their head and shoulders raised and their body inclined over toward the injured side, keeping the injured lung lowermost. This will allow the uninjured lung to function without restriction and will help keep it free of collecting blood;
- loosen any tight clothing which restricts breathing;
- if possible, place the arm on the injured side in an elevation sling;
- if the casualty becomes unconscious, place them into the recovery position keeping the injured side lowermost;
- monitor breathing and circulation and resuscitate if necessary;
- call for an ambulance.

Penetrating Chest Wound

This type of injury can cause serious problems with the normal mechanism of breathing and is very serious.

Every time the casualty tries to breathe in, the resulting vacuum inside the chest can suck air in through the hole in the chest wall (sucking wound). This air collects inside the chest cavity, but not inside the lung. It collects in the space between the outside of the lung and the inside of the chest wall (pleural space). As the air and blood from the injury collects in the chest cavity, it makes the lung begin to collapse.

Recognition

- A history of impact with a sharp or penetrating object. The penetrating object may be visible.
- The wound may bubble with blood and the sound of air sucking in through the hole may be heard.
- Laboured and distressed breathing.
- The chest wall on the injured side may not move when the casualty breathes in.
- Signs and symptoms of shock may be present, including blueness of the extremities.
- Coughing up blood, which is often bright red and frothy.

Treatment

The main aim of treatment is to prevent any further air getting in through the hole and treat the casualty for the resulting shock.

- Expose the wound and immediately make a temporary seal over it with the palm of the casualty's hand. If the casualty cannot assist, use your own hand.
- Make a more permanent seal over the hole with a sterile wound dressing from the first aid kit. Use a large wound dressing for this to ensure that the tails are long enough to wrap around the chest. Ensure that the applied dressing is making an airtight seal over the wound.
- Do not attempt to remove the object if it is protruding from the wound. If possible, stop it from moving around and seal the wound around the edges.
- Rest the casualty in the position which best helps their breathing: ideally, inclined with the injured side lowermost.
- Treat for shock where possible.
- If the casualty becomes unconscious, put them into the recovery position, keeping the injured side lowermost.
- Monitor breathing and circulation and resuscitate if necessary.
- Call for an ambulance.

Internal Chest Injury

Internal chest injury can be caused by:

- fractured ribs;
- penetrating chest wounds;
- the immense pressure of air generated from an explosion (shock wave).

Recognition

- History of the accident.
- The casualty may complain of chest pain even though there may be no visible damage to the chest wall.
- Laboured and distressed breathing.
- The chest wall on the injured side may not move when the casualty breathes in.
- Signs and symptoms of shock may be present, including blueness of the extremities.
- Coughing up blood, which is often bright red and frothy.

Treatment

- Rest the casualty in the position which best helps their breathing. This is often laid down with their head and shoulders raised and their body inclined over toward the injured side, keeping the injured lung lowermost. This will allow the uninjured lung to function without restriction and will help keep it free of collecting blood.
- Loosen any tight clothing which restricts breathing.
- If there is evidence of fractured ribs or a penetrating wound treat accordingly (see above).
- If the casualty becomes unconscious, place them into the recovery position keeping the injured side lowermost.
- Monitor breathing and circulation and resuscitate if necessary.
- Call for an ambulance.

Abdominal Injuries

The abdominal cavity contains many important organs and structures. All abdominal injuries have the potential to become life-threatening.

In general, abdominal injuries fall into two categories: open wounds and closed (blunt) injuries.

Injuries to the abdomen have two potential effects, both of which can be life-threatening.

1. Shock, resulting from internal and external blood loss.
2. Infection. This can be introduced into the abdomen by a penetrating object, or spread from internal organs such as the intestine when it is perforated.

Open Abdominal Injuries

Penetrating wounds to the abdomen, such as stab wounds, are often much more serious than they first appear. Although the visible wound may only be small, the damage inside the cavity is often extensive. In some cases, abdominal organs may protrude from the wound.

Recognition

- History of impact or violence to the abdomen.
- Visible blood loss. Remember, this may only be a small amount compared to the internal bleeding.
- Internal organs may be visible protruding from the wound.
- Shock. In many cases this is severe.

Treatment

- Lay the casualty down and reassure them.
- If the wound goes across the abdomen, raise the casualty's knees and place padding as support underneath them. This position often increases the comfort of the casualty and stops the wound from gaping open.

  If the wound goes down the abdomen, lay the casualty flat to prevent the wound from gaping open.
- Cover the wound with a large, sterile wound dressing. Do not bandage it in place too tightly as this may cause further pain and damage.

X If there is an object penetrating into the abdomen, do not remove it. Gently support it to stop it moving around and bandage gently around the edges where it penetrates.

X Do not try to push any protruding organs back inside the abdomen. Cover them with the sterile dressing.

- If the casualty coughs or vomits, gently press onto the dressing. This may help prevent the abdominal organs from pushing out of the wound.
- Treat the casualty for shock, and keep them as still as possible.
- If the casualty becomes unconscious, place them into the recovery position and monitor breathing. Provide support to the injured area during the turning process.
- Call for an ambulance.

Closed Abdominal injuries

These are caused by blunt impact to the abdomen. In many cases it is very easy to underestimate the severity of the condition if the internal injury is hidden from view.

Recognition

- History of impact or violence to the abdomen.
- The casualty may complain of pain and tenderness at the site of injury.
- Signs and symptoms of shock may be present (see section 11).
- The casualty may have difficulty in breathing. In some cases, the impact may have severely winded the casualty or caused damage to the diaphragm muscle.

Treatment

- Reassure the casualty and lay them down in the most comfortable position possible. This is often on the back with the head, shoulders and knees raised and supported.
- Treat the casualty for shock.
- If the casualty becomes unconscious, place them into the recovery position and monitor airway, breathing and circulation.
- Call for an ambulance.

Head Injuries

Although preventable, injuries to the head are common in many working environments and in some cases they can be very serious.

The brain is situated inside the skull for protection, and as we have already seen, it is one of the most important organs of the body. The function of the brain is to control and co-ordinate the majority of body functions. Injuries to the head can cause temporary or permanent damage to the brain which can have a widespread and sometimes life-threatening effect.

Concussion

This is a temporary and reversible disturbance of the brain's normal function. It occurs when the brain moves or 'shakes' inside the skull and is usually caused by a blow to the head or jaw.

Recognition

Concussion can occur without causing unconsciousness, or in some cases the duration of unconsciousness may have been so brief that the casualty cannot remember the initial accident.

- History of a blow to, or shaking of, the head.
- There may be some disturbance in normal vision.
- The casualty may feel nauseous or may vomit.
- Possible dizziness or giddiness.
- The casualty may complain of a headache.
- There may be a partial loss of memory, particularly of the events immediately before the accident.
- Possible unconsciousness, usually of short duration

Treatment

In most cases, the treatment of concussion only involves rest and monitoring the casualty for any deterioration (as a reversible condition it should go away on its own). In all cases, however, the casualty must be advised to see their doctor after work or if any symptoms are persistent or become worse.

- Keep the casualty at rest and reassure them.
- If necessary, carry out the treatment for the unconscious casualty and call for an ambulance.
- If there is a lump or bump developing on the head, apply a cold compress to reduce swelling.
- Monitor the casualty for signs and symptoms which may indicate cerebral compression, even if the casualty has apparently recovered.
- If the casualty suffered unconsciousness, even for a short period, arrange for them to be taken to hospital for further examination and observation.
- If any signs or symptoms are still present, or the casualty feels at all unwell, arrange for them to be taken to hospital for further examination and observation.
- If all signs and all symptoms have gone, the casualty may return to work but keep an eye on them and tell them to report back to you if any symptoms recur or they begin to feel unwell. Remember though, the casualty must still be advised to see their doctor after work.

X DO NOT let the casualty lie down or sleep in the first aid or rest room following concussion. It is much harder to spot deterioration in the condition when the casualty is asleep. If the casualty is unable to sit up due to the severity of the concussion, they should go to hospital immediately.

Compression of the Brain

This is due to a build up of pressure within the skull. The pressure is exerted onto the brain and seriously interferes with its ability to control and co-ordinate the functions of the body. It can result in permanent damage to the brain.

Pressure can build up inside the skull for a variety of reasons including medical conditions such as tumours, injuries such as bleeding from blood vessels inside the skull or depressed fractures of the skull.

The onset of compression is not always sudden, and it can develop some hours or even days after a head injury. This is why observations on a casualty who has suffered concussion are so important.

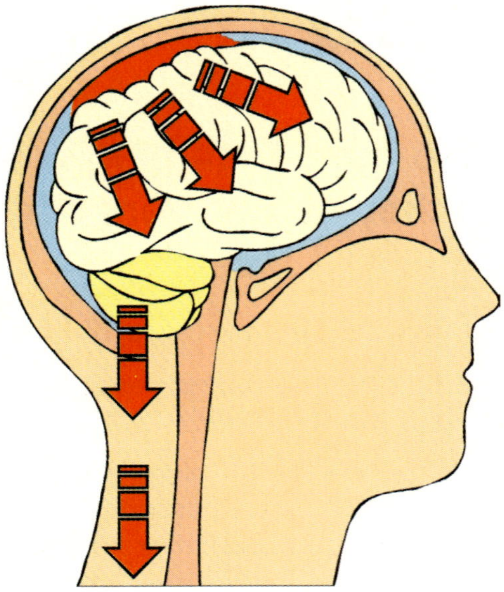

Fig.42 Compression Injury

Recognition

As the condition develops, the signs and symptoms become more and more pronounced.

- History of an unusual, persistent headache or history of impact to the head.
- In the initial stages, the signs and symptoms of concussion may be present.
- As the compression develops, the casualty's level of response will deteriorate. In most cases this will result in unconsciousness.
- While the casualty remains conscious, a weakness or paralysis of one side of the body may develop.
- Breathing may become laboured, noisy and irregular.
- The pulse rate may slow down and become strong and irregular.
- The pupils may be different sizes, and their reaction to light may become slow or absent.
- The casualty's skin temperature may rise, and his face may become flushed and warm to the touch. This is due to a rise in blood pressure.

Treatment

There is nothing that the first aider can do to release the pressure building up inside the skull so treatment revolves around A.B.C.

- If the casualty is conscious, place and support them in a comfortable position, preferably with the head and shoulders slightly raised.
- Treat any other injuries, such as bleeding from a scalp wound.
- If the casualty is unconscious, place in recovery position and ensure the airway remains open and clear.
- Carry out resuscitation if necessary.
- Call for an ambulance as soon as possible.

Bleeding from the Scalp

The scalp has a very good blood supply which helps in the body's heat control mechanism. Although high in number, the blood vessels in the scalp are relatively small and therefore controlling bleeding is usually easy.

Treatment

- Rest and reassure the casualty.
- Examine the wound for any obvious embedded object.
- Control the bleeding with gentle pressure, using a sterile wound dressing.
- If the wound is large or the bleeding will not stop, arrange for them to be taken to hospital for further treatment.
- Monitor for signs of concussion and treat accordingly.

Test Your Knowledge

1) A casualty received a sudden blow to the head 2 minutes ago. He briefly lost consciousness but now says that he feels sick and a little dizzy, though he seems to be improving.

   a) What condition is he likely to be suffering from? ....

   b) What will happen to the following if compression is suspected?

   Pulse .... Breathing .... Skin ....

2) The correct position in which to put a casualty who has a head injury who is

   a) conscious is .... and

   b) unconscious is ....

Eye Injuries

Although not usually life-threatening, eye injuries can easily result in serious, even permanent damage. Delay in diagnosis and treatment can often lead to the injury worsening.

The eye is a very delicate organ and very susceptible to injury and infection. To help understand eye injuries and what could go wrong with the eye, the first aider needs a basic knowledge of the anatomy of the eye.

The eye is supported and protected inside a bony socket in the skull (the orbit). Inside the orbit, the eye has a good range of movement which is provided by muscles. The eye is constantly bathed in a mild solution of salt in water (tears) which lubricates eye movement. When the upper eye lid moves (e.g. during the process of blinking), it cleans and lubricates the surface of the front of the eye.

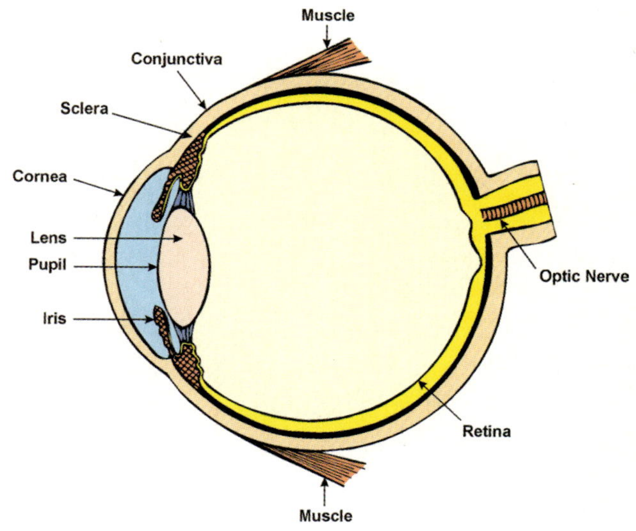

Fig.43. The Eye

The Sclera

This is a tough, white, opaque membrane which helps maintain the shape of the eye.

The Cornea

This is the front part of the sclera. It is transparent and therefore allows light to enter the eye.

The Iris

This is a coloured membrane which has a central aperture or hole called the pupil. The pupil opens and closes in response to light, and its purpose is to help regulate the amount of light passing through to the lens.

The Lens

This clear disc changes in shape and thickness and focuses the light into a clear image on the retina.

The Retina

This is the light-sensitive lining of the inner eye. It is comprised of nerve cells which convert the focused light image into electrical impulses.

The Optic Nerve

This is a bundle of nerve fibres along which electrical impulses from the retina pass to the brain.

A large proportion of injuries sustained in the workplace involve the eyes, mainly from foreign objects, but also from chemical splashes or vapours, intense light or infection. Injuries are commonest in occupations which involve turning, spinning, drilling, hammering, grinding and welding. It has been estimated that one third of all eye injuries treated in hospitals are sustained at work.

Because the eye is such a delicate organ, first aiders must treat any injury or condition of the eye with extreme care. Failure to do so could easily make the injury worse, resulting in disastrous consequences for the casualty's comfort and vision.

A first aider should know how to examine the eye of a casualty and, from that examination, be able to determine what injury is present, decide on appropriate treatment and whether the casualty requires further medical assistance.

Examining the Eye

Before examination:

- The casualty should be encouraged not to rub the eyes.
- If possible, you should wash your hands.
- If the casualty is wearing contact lenses, they should be advised to remove them if possible.
- Sit the casualty down in an area with good lighting and facing the source of light.
- Stand behind the casualty and support their head against your body.

- Tilt the casualty's head well back. Hold the eye open with the thumb and index finger of the hand on the side of the eye being examined. This may be very uncomfortable for the casualty so be careful and give plenty of reassurance. Always explain what you are going to do and do not make any sudden or unexpected movements. Do not hurry the process.
- With the eye now held open, inspect the front visible part of the eye.
- Ask the casualty to look up, down, left and right so the whole of the exposed eye surface can be examined.
- Observe carefully for foreign objects:
  - on the front of the eyeball;
  - on the white part of the eye;
  - on the part inside the lower eye lid.

The object may be seen to be:

- glistening or black;
- moving (in which case the first aider may attempt removal);
- fixed or embedded (in which case the first aider must not attempt removal).

X DO NOT attempt to fold back or examine under the upper lid. This is a potentially dangerous technique and should only be carried out by a qualified and experienced person.

Overall, the eye may be:

- Painful.
- Red and swollen (this is usually due to the casualty rubbing it).
- Watering.

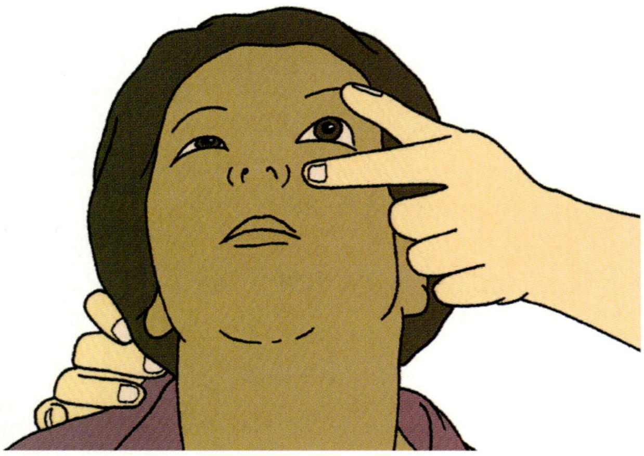

Fig.44. Examining the Eye

In some cases, the casualty may not allow the first aider to attempt examination, or the first aider may not feel confident enough to perform the procedure. If this is the case, simply apply an eye pad over the injured eye and seek further medical aid. Do not risk further injury or discomfort.

Foreign Objects

Small foreign objects such as dust, grit and even loose eyelashes can cause considerable irritation when they touch the sensitive front part of the eyeball. In some cases, especially when the casualty has been rubbing the affected eye, the foreign object may scratch the cornea. This scratch will not be visible to the first aider during the examination procedure.

If, on examination, a foreign object cannot be seen but there is still persistent pain, irritation and watering, it may help to irrigate or wash the eye.

Routine Eye Wash

This technique involves flushing the eye to remove the object. Ideally, a sterile eye-wash solution should be used, but fresh water decanted from a very clean glass or similar receptacle will suffice.

- Explain the procedure to the casualty.
- Ensure the container to be used is free from dirt and dust and if using a sterile eye-wash, check that it is within the expiry date. Also check that the seal on the container is unbroken.
- Position the casualty as for examining the eye but also incline the head toward the affected side. This will ensure that the irrigation fluid will drain away over the side of the face and not contaminate the unaffected eye.
- Give the casualty a towel or other absorbent material to hold by the side of the face to soak up the irrigation liquid as it drains away.
- Open the affected eye in the same way as for examining the eye and gently commence irrigation into the inner (nose side) corner of the eye.

The casualty is likely to flinch as the liquid touches the eye, so be prepared for this. To help control the flinching:

- Explain what you are doing to the casualty and get them to take a few deep breaths and relax.
- Allow a few drops of liquid to drip onto the casualty's cheek below the eye, then move the flow to the inner corner.

- Keeping the eye open, gently allow the liquid to flow into the inner corner of the eye and across the surface. This should continue for 10 to 15 seconds and then gently dry off the area without rubbing.
- If irritation persists, repeat the process once more.

- If the object will not wash out or if irritation persists, even though the object has been flushed away, gently cover the affected eye with an eye pad and ensure the casualty is taken to further medical aid.

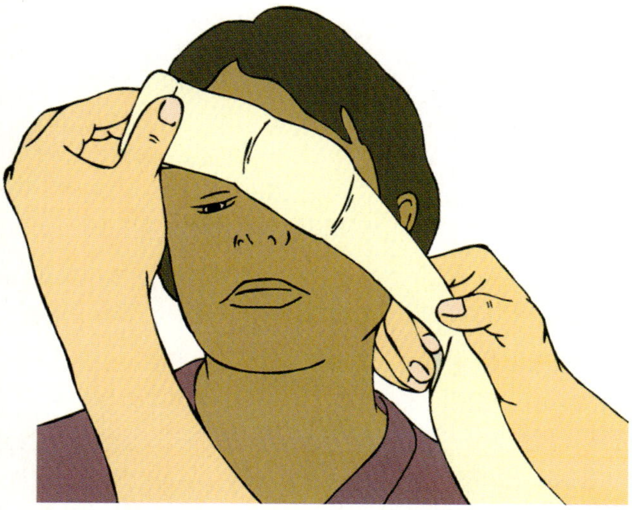

Fig.45. The Eye Pad

Embedded Foreign Objects

If the eye has been penetrated by an object such as a fragment of glass or splinter of metal, it is a very serious injury and, although not usually life-threatening, it can certainly be sight-threatening.

- On examination, the object may be visible if it protrudes from the surface.
- Intense pain, although if the object is small and the object does not protrude from the surface, the pain may not develop until some time after the injury has occurred.
- The casualty may be in a high state of distress and panic.
- If the eyeball has been penetrated, there may be blood or a watery fluid leaking from the wound.

Treatment may be made all the more difficult due to the high state of distress and panic.

- Lay the casualty down and reassure them. Impress on them the importance that they remain calm and do not let them rub the eye.
- DO NOT attempt to remove the embedded object.
- Gently and lightly cover **both eyes** with sterile eye pads to help reduce movement of the eyes and reduce any irritation from light.
- If the embedded object is long and protrudes out from the eye, a built up dressing which does not apply pressure to the object should be applied.
- The casualty should be transported to hospital by ambulance. If they are encouraged to walk, the eyes will move and make the injury worse.

Chemical Splashes in the Eye

Chemicals can cause serious and possibly permanent damage to the eye. Most chemicals will cause burns which can be very painful.

- There may be evidence of a chemical or container at the scene of the accident and the casualty may be able to tell you what has happened.
- Intense pain.
- The eye may become red and swollen.
- Excessive watering of the eye.
- The eye may be tightly closed and the casualty may not be able to open it.

Treatment must be quick and effective. If the chemical is not removed it will continue to burn, causing more damage.

In extreme cases, especially where the casualty is in a high state of distress or panic, it may be necessary to get others at the scene to help with treatment.

The aim of treatment is to fully wash the eye to disperse the chemical and cool down the burn.

- Circumstances will dictate whether the casualty should be laying down or bending over a sink or built-in eye-wash station. The irrigation must be carried out by the quickest method possible.
- Reassure the casualty and try to calm them down.
- Carry out emergency eye irrigation as follows:
    - Lie the casualty down, with the head inclined toward the injured side

      OR
    - Lean the casualty over a sink with the head turned so the affected eye is downward.
    - Hold the head still, open the affected eye and flood the area with gently running fresh water or, if available, an emergency eye-wash solution.
    - Being careful not to spread contamination to unaffected areas, continue irrigation for at least 20 minutes and ensure that the irrigation fluid reaches under both the upper and lower lids of the eye.
- When irrigation is complete, cover the eye with a sterile eye pad and take the casualty to further medical aid immediately. If possible, send details of the chemical with the casualty.

Glass in the Eye

Fragments of glass in the eye can be very difficult

to see and are likely to cut the surface of the eye. First aiders should not try to remove glass from the eye, whether embedded or not. Treat the casualty as for an embedded object and call for an ambulance.

Conjunctivitis

This condition occurs when the membrane which covers the front of the eye and inner sides of the eye lids (the conjunctiva) becomes inflamed and swollen. It can be caused by germs, pollen, dust and chemical fumes, or infection.

- The casualty will often feel a pricking sensation or irritation in the eye without any obvious history of a foreign object.
- The eye may become red, swollen and may begin to water.

There is very little treatment which a first aider can give for this condition.

- A routine eye irrigation may soothe the eye and relieve irritation for a short time.
- The casualty should be advised to see their own doctor or be taken to hospital for further examination and treatment.
- The first aider should wash their hands carefully after contact with the casualty and should avoid touching any eyes that may be infected.

Blows to the Eye

Severe blows to the eye can cause serious damage to the light sensitive lining of the eye (the retina) and other internal structures. The severity of this type of injury is often underestimated.

In all cases of a blow to the eye which causes pain and impaired vision:

- Place the casualty at rest.
- Cover both eyes with sterile eye pads.
- Arrange removal to hospital by ambulance.
- The first aider should wash their hands carefully after contact with the casualty and should avoid touching any eyes that may be infected.

Welders Flash (Arc-Eye)

This condition follows exposure of the unprotected eye to the intense light produced during gas or electric welding and cutting. Welding operators are usually aware of the risks and use protective shields to prevent injury. The main risk is usually to others who are working in the area who have no such protection. The intense light can cause serious damage to the retina, and in some cases may even burn a permanent image onto it, even from a distance of 200 feet. The longer the exposure, the more severe the injury will be.

The casualty may not complain of any symptoms until some time after exposure. There may be:

- Intense burning or irritation in the eye. Many people have described a sensation similar to having grains of sand in the eye.
- Reddening and watering of the eye.
- Impaired vision, usually with a permanent 'blind spot' in the centre of the field of vision.
- In serious cases, total vision may be lost.

The aim of treatment is simply to prevent the condition worsening.

- Rest and reassure the casualty.
- If pain is severe, gently irrigate the eye with a sterile eye-wash solution or fresh water. Alternatively, gently apply a cold compress.
- Cover the affected eye with a sterile eye pad.
- Take the casualty to further medical aid for further examination and treatment.

Remember!

All eye injuries are potentially serious and are liable to give rise to further complications such as corneal scratch and infection.

If ever in doubt as to the severity of an eye injury, seek further medical advice from your occupational health department, general practitioner or local hospital casualty department.

Test Your Knowledge

1) What is the treatment for someone who has splashed bleach into his eyes?

....

2) Why is a visit to a hospital casualty department recommended for all eye incidents which cause concern to the casualty?

....

Poisons and Harmful Substances

Many chemicals used in the workplace can have a detrimental effect on a person's health. Every first aider should be familiar with the chemicals specific to their place of work.

Within industry, a vast quantity and variety of chemicals are used. Many of these chemicals are hazardous, from common cleaning products and solvents used by the smallest business to large amounts of highly toxic substances used by manufacturing and processing plants. This means that every employee may be at some level of risk whilst at work.

Chemical substances may affect the body in many ways. Some may be corrosive, causing burns to the skin, eyes or lungs. Others can be taken into the body through the skin, by inhalation or through the digestive system, and eventually end up in the blood stream where they can affect the whole of the body, especially the function of the brain (systemic).

The harmful effects of some chemicals may develop over a long period of time causing illness and disability. Others, however, present a more immediate danger, where even brief exposure can prove fatal.

The subject of harmful substances and poisons is huge, and in general well beyond the scope of this manual and certainly beyond the range of knowledge a first aider can be expected to learn. However, first aiders must be aware of the dangers within their own particular workplace and be familiar with the chemicals and harmful substances which are relevant to the workplace environment in which they practise first aid.

Hazard Data Sheets

Chemical manufacturers and suppliers issue hazard data sheets or COSHH sheets (Control Of Substances Hazardous to Health) for all the hazardous substances they provide to employers. These sheets give up-to-date information about the substance such as what it is, how it should be used, the conditions under which it should be stored and used, protective equipment which should be worn when using it and lots more. Good data sheets will also provide medical information relevant to the substance such as how it may enter the body, the signs and symptoms it may produce and, most importantly, emergency first aid and advanced medical treatments which may be required. The hazard data sheet should be displayed where the chemical is being used and it is recommended that all first aiders in the workplace are familiar with the location and content of their company's sheets. If in doubt, ask your manager or supervisor for further information.

Chemical Poisoning

Poisonous substances taken into the body in sufficient quantity may have temporary or permanent effects. If the substance enters the blood stream, it will be carried to all parts of the body which may result in a generalised effect. In some cases, the harmful substance may cause damage to the blood itself, preventing the blood cells from carrying oxygen to other body cells. On reaching the brain, the substance may cause widespread generalised effects, which can result in unconsciousness and even the stoppage of breathing and circulation.

Routes of entry into the body

There are four main routes of entry for poisons and harmful substances into the body.

- Inhalation (breathed in)
- Ingestion (swallowed)
- Absorbed (through the skin)
- Injected (through the skin)

Recognition

Because there are so many different poisons and harmful substances which can affect the body, it is not possible in the text of this manual to give specific signs and symptoms, but the following list are perhaps most common. Some of the recognition points may depend on the type of substances and the route of entry into the body.

- History. There may be evidence or clues of harmful substances at the scene or perhaps a bystander can give you information relating to the cause.

- Breathing difficulty and perhaps coughing.
- Headache.
- Delirium and confusion.
- Skin burns and blisters (corrosives).
- Skin rashes and skin irritation.
- Nausea and vomiting.
- Aches and pains.
- Diarrhoea.
- The eyes may redden and begin to water.
- Muscular twitching and convulsions.
- Unconsciousness.
- Respiratory and cardiac arrest.

Treatment

Again, due to the large number of harmful substances, it is not possible to be specific about treatments and the following points reflect a general overview of treatments.

When **Inhaled.**

Gas vapours and fumes from solvents may be inhaled, causing irritation to the lungs and respiratory distress.

Examples of inhaled substances are smoke fumes, carbon monoxide, fumes from solvents and cleaning solutions and spirit-based solutions such as paint and white spirit.

- Do not become a casualty yourself. Remember, specialist breathing equipment may be required to enter a contaminated area.
- Remove the casualty from the contaminated area, and if possible into a fresh air environment. In some cases, rescue may have to be performed by properly equipped personnel.
- Place the casualty in a position which best facilitates breathing and loosen any tight or restrictive clothing.
- Carry out the A.B.C. checks and treat accordingly. If the casualty is unconscious, place them into the recovery position.
- If appropriate, follow any specific information given on the hazard data sheet.
- Ensure an ambulance has been called and pass on details of the harmful substance to the ambulance crew on arrival.

When **Absorbed.**

Certain chemicals can easily absorb through the skin and enter the blood stream.

Examples of absorbed substances are spirit-based solutions such as petrol and white spirit, and insecticides.

- Do not become a casualty yourself. If necessary, wear protective clothing to prevent cross-contamination (gloves, goggles and apron).
- Sit the casualty down and keep them at rest.
- Carefully remove any contaminated clothing being careful not to spread contamination to unaffected areas. In some cases, it may be more beneficial to cut clothing away.
- Rinse the chemical off the skin with copious amounts of water, again being careful not to spread contamination.
- If appropriate, place the casualty in the recovery position or resuscitate if necessary.
- Follow any specific information given on the hazard data sheet.
- Ensure an ambulance has been called and pass on details of the harmful substance to the ambulance crew on arrival.

When **Ingested.**

Swallowed substances may cause stomach and bowel irritation resulting in nausea, vomiting and painful abdominal cramps. If the substance is corrosive, it may cause burns to the lips, mouth and throat leading to airway obstruction.

- Sit the casualty down and keep them at rest. This will help slow down the speed of absorption into the blood stream.
- If the lips, mouth or throat are burned and the casualty is conscious, give frequent sips of cold water to cool the area, reduce swelling and dilute the chemical.
- DO NOT make the casualty vomit as this can increase the burning effect in the mouth and throat and may block the airway.
- If appropriate, place the casualty in the recovery position or resuscitate if necessary.
- Follow any specific information given on the hazard data sheet.
- Ensure an ambulance has been called and pass on details of the swallowed substance (e.g. when taken, how much taken) to the ambulance crew on arrival. Also pass on any empty bottles or containers which could provide important information.

When **Injected.**

Harmful substances can be injected into the body through the skin.

A harmful substance may also enter through a puncture wound caused by a contaminated sharp object, and even an animal bite.

- Do not become a casualty yourself. Take care not to expose yourself to the sharp object.
- Sit the casualty down and at rest. If the substance has been injected into muscle and soft tissue, movement and agitation of the injection site may increase absorption into the blood stream.
- If appropriate, place the casualty in the recovery position or resuscitate if necessary.
- Follow any specific information given on the hazard data sheet.
- Ensure an ambulance has been called and, if possible, pass on details of the substance to the ambulance crew on arrival.

Stings and Bites

Although syringes and hypodermic needles are perhaps the most obvious cause of injected poisons, by far the most common are insect and plant stings. These can occur in any workplace, particularly in the summertime.

As well as following the main principles already detailed, and cooling the reddened, swelling area, you need to:

- be watchful for anaphylactic shock (see appendix F.1) and deal with it appropriately
- if the sting is protruding from the skin, gently flick it away using you index finger and thumb – do not squeeze it
- get medical help if the swelling is inside the mouth or on the neck as this may obstruct breathing
- be prepared to give rescue breaths, if necessary
- do NOT apply creams or sprays to the area, in case of allergies
- use cold water to reduce the swelling
- reassure the casualty and treat for shock, as necessary.

If the casualty has suffered an animal bite, treat it as a wound. Carefully wash it without rubbing, cover with a sterile dressing and ensure medical help.

In summary, the main aim in all cases of contamination with poisonous and harmful substances is :

- Prevent or reduce further contamination.
- Maintain an adequate open airway.
- Resuscitate the casualty if necessary.
- Seek urgent medical aid.

And remember, information relating to harmful substances for your own workplace can be found on your company's hazard data sheets. Ensure you are familiar with their location and content.

Test Your Knowledge

1) Certain chemicals require specific treatment. Where would you find the details of this specific treatment?

....

2) When dealing with a first aid incident at work where chemicals or poisons have been involved what are the main aims of treatment (please tick one answer):

   a) Dilute with water, obtain safety data sheet, treat as necessary, send to hospital.
   b) Remove from the source, protect the airway, resuscitate if necessary and get emergency aid.
   c) Identify the source, place in the recovery position, treat for shock, get emergency aid.
   d) Find the COSHH leaflet, treat as necessary, monitor, and get help.

Blast Injuries

It is very rare for a first aider to have to deal with injuries resulting from a blast, but if the specific risk exists in the workplace, the first aider must be prepared for the worst.

Some places of work contain items which have a specific risk of explosion. Apart from the obvious explosive compounds such as gunpowder and fuel, any piece of pressurised workplace equipment has a potential to explode. Examples are gas cylinders, sterilising autoclaves, pressurised hydraulic systems and air compressors.

The effects of blast injury on the body can be devastating. This is mainly due to the combined effects of multiple injuries. There are four main elements of an explosion, each with its own characteristics and potential for injury.

1. Light flash.

   Some types of explosion may emit an intense light. Although it only lasts for a fraction of a second, it can be bright enough to cause considerable damage to the light-sensitive lining of the eye in the form of a burn, very similar to that of welder's flash (see section 18).

2. Pressure wave.

   As an explosion occurs, the surrounding air is compressed at an immense speed. This huge compressed air flow (or shock wave) can cause considerable damage to cavities of the body, in particular the chest and middle ear. In the case of the chest, it can result in serious internal bleeding from damaged blood vessels. In the case of the ear, it can result in a constant, loud ringing in the ear (tinnitus) or even rupture the ear-drum.

3. Fragmentation.

   The shock wave emitting from the blast is often powerful enough to propel debris through the air. This debris is often in the form of small, sharp objects which can embed deep into body tissue, causing serious internal and external bleeding.

4. Heat.

   In many cases of explosion, there is an element of heat involved which emits from the source of explosion. This heat can be intense enough to cause extensive flash burns to any exposed area of the skin, which often includes the neck and face.

Management of Blast Injury

Although there may be different types of injury to different parts of the body, it is essential that the ABC principle is followed. The individual treatments for all injuries are detailed elsewhere in this manual.

Airway

- Ensure that it is clear and open.
- If unconscious, place into the recovery position (see section 9).
- Cool any burns around the neck and face to reduce swelling (see section 12).

Breathing

- Treat any injury to the chest and ensure that, if possible, the casualty is placed with the injured side of the chest lowermost (see section 15).
- Resuscitate if necessary (see section 8).
- If toxic or harmful fumes have been inhaled, try to ensure a good, fresh air supply for the casualty (see section 19).

Circulation

- Control any bleeding from open wounds, using a built-up dressing technique around any embedded objects. If there are multiple open wounds, deal first with those which are bleeding the most (see section 10).
- Cool down any burns and cover them to prevent infection (see section 12).
- Treat the casualty for shock (see section 11).

Other Treatments

- If the casualty has sustained a light flash to the eyes, treat as for welder's flash (see section 18).
- If the casualty has sustained damage to the ear, or has any hearing impairment, cover the ears with sterile dressings.
- Reassure the casualty at all times. Being involved in an explosion is a particularly frightening experience for all concerned.
- Call for an ambulance and, if necessary, other emergency services.

General Illness at Work

As a first aider, you may find that you spend just as much time dealing with people who don't feel well as you do dealing with people who have injuries.

It is important that the first aider is aware of the actions which should be taken when presented with illnesses at work, remembering that the ill person needs to be safe as a result of your treatment.

Serious medical conditions which can come on suddenly and may constitute a medical emergency such as asthma, heart conditions, stroke, diabetes and epilepsy are covered in the appendix of this manual.

Common, and more minor, illnesses which may occur at work include headache, toothache, earache, stomach-ache/nausea and cold/influenza.

Many common ailments may be relieved by proprietary drugs which can be bought over the counter from a chemist or other outlet. The decision to take these medicines is the responsibility of the person suffering the ailment and is outside the responsibility of the first aider. **It is stressed that under no circumstances should a first aider advise an ill person to take, or actually dispense, any medication whatsoever at work.** This could land you and your company in big trouble!

In some cases of illness at work, the person may have suffered from the illness before, and may even be taking medication prescribed by their doctor. If this is the case, the ill person will know when, and how, to take such medication.

General Points when Dealing with Illness at Work

It must be remembered that people at work are of adult age, and therefore capable of making decisions for themselves with regard to their condition and what action should be taken.

- A first aider is not expected to be able to make a true diagnosis of the underlying illness (this is a doctor's job). However, the first aider is expected to be able to make a common-sense decision about their overall condition and what action should be taken next.
- If possible, deal with the person in a quiet, private area such as the first-aid room.
- Always listen carefully and sympathetically to any history or symptoms which the person tells you.
- Whether you have an idea or not of what may be the cause of the problem, never have any doubt about someone who is ill at work. Get qualified medical help rather than hope for the best.
- In many cases, the only treatment that a first aider can give for an illness is advice.
    - If the person feels well enough to return to work, and at their request, they may do so. However, it is good practice for the first aider to look in on the person from time to time throughout the day to check on their condition. The casualty should always be advised to see their doctor should the condition persist or worsen.
    - If, in their own opinion, the person is too ill to return to work, at their request they may wish to go home. If this is the case, the first aider should ensure that the chosen method of transportation home will be safe, bearing in mind their illness. For example, a casualty who is having bad migraine which is causing disturbances in their vision and concentration should not be allowed to drive themselves home.
    - If any person is too ill to continue work, they are ill enough to warrant seeing their doctor. Bearing this in mind, the first aider should always advise the casualty to see their doctor as soon as possible. If they don't take your advice, that is their decision.
- If the nature of the illness is such that it could spread from person to person (communicable), the casualty should not be allowed to continue work and should be advised to see their doctor immediately. If they remain at work, it could put other members of staff at risk and will not allow for rest, which is an important factor in their recovery. Examples of common communicable illness are influenza, and diarrhoea/vomiting.
- If a person is unable to continue work due to an illness, inform their supervisor or manager at the earliest possible opportunity.

- It is advisable that all occurrences of illness at work are formally recorded.
  - It will confirm that the illness was dealt with correctly by the first aider and provide a written record of any advice which was given.
  - It will allow management to review occurrences of illness at work and evaluate the potential of the working environment causing or contributing towards the illness.

The Particular Needs of Female Colleagues

There are a few conditions which could develop at work which are unique to female members of staff. Two common conditions are painful periods (dysmenorrhoea) and problems during pregnancy.

- It is often best that a female first aider deals with this nature of problem.
- Always be discreet, offering privacy and rest.
- The person themselves are usually the best judge of their needs, so listen to them carefully.
- If there is any suspicion that the discomfort being experienced is not usual or normal, seek further medical aid.

Mental Distress

If you notice unusual behaviour such as irritability or aggression, or bouts of uncontrollable weeping, it may be an indication of mental distress.

Your colleague needs to seek medical help and may need quietness, support, time and encouragement to get help.

If you are worried about your colleague, you may need to arrange for them to go to hospital. Make sure that somebody else drives you there.

Test Your Knowledge

1) Name six signs or symptoms which could help you in your diagnosis of any illness/injury:

i ....

ii ....

iii ....

iv ....

v ....

vi ....

Moving a Casualty

Under certain circumstances, a casualty may have to be moved. It is important that a first aider has a good understanding of when this may be necessary and how to do it safely.

First aiders should never attempt to move or lift a casualty, except in the most extreme of emergencies. Where there is no danger at the scene of the accident to the casualty or first aider, the casualty should remain where they are until expert help arrives.

If a workplace has difficult or restricted access, the risk assessment should take this into consideration and, where necessary, provide mechanical aids for the lifting and movement of injured people, such as a 'carry chair'. Additional training will be required for anyone responsible for using such specialised equipment.

There are four main situations that can be regarded as true emergencies and which may require a casualty to be immediately removed from danger. In such cases, the rescuers must consider the risks to themselves - remember, do not become a casualty yourself!

- Danger from a collapsing building or falling object.
- An area that is on fire or filling with smoke or other harmful gases and fumes.
- In water where the casualty is in danger of drowning.
- Danger from explosion or firearms.

In an emergency, and where the manual handling of injured people is necessary, the following guidelines should be adhered to:

- **Avoid lifting**
  - whenever possible, do not lift;
  - encourage people to help themselves;
  - make use of available equipment and lifting aids.

- **If lifting is unavoidable:**
  - assess the task:
    - what are you going to do?
    - why is it necessary?
    - what are the difficulties and constraints?
  - assess the casualty:
    - how heavy are they?
    - what is their ability with regard to communication and helping themselves ?
    - what physical and behavioural constraints are there, including injuries?
  - the environment:
    - location and conditions
    - the distance and route to be travelled
    - availability of help and specialised equipment
  - yourself:
    - level of skill
    - fitness and ability
    - clothing

Making the Lift

- Get someone to help you if possible - 'many hands make light work'.
- Keep the weight as close to yourself as possible.
- Keep the feet placed a shoulder width apart to ensure good balance.
- Bend the knees and keep the back straight.
- Avoid twisting and stooping.
- Raise your head as you start to lift.
- Lift with the power of the leg muscles, not the back.

Transportation Methods

The Human Crutch Method

This method can be used if the casualty is conscious and able to walk with some assistance.

- If available, give the casualty a walking aid.
- Stand on the weakest or injured side of the casualty.

- Pass the casualty's arm around your neck and grasp their hand or wrist with your hand.
- Place your other arm around the casualty's waist and grasp hold of their belt or clothing for extra support.
- Taking small steps, move off with the inside foot. Allow the pace to be governed by the casualty.
- Offer continual encouragement and reassurance to the casualty.

The Drag Method

This method should only be used in an emergency, to move a casualty who is unconscious or unable to walk. The method described should not be used if there are injuries to the head or neck or back (although if the casualty is unconscious, this may be difficult to determine).

- Squat behind the casualty and assist them to sit up with their arms crossed over their chest.
- Place your arms under the casualty's armpits and grasp their wrists.
- Carefully, whilst squat walking backwards, drag the casualty clear.

If the casualty is wearing a coat or jacket, it may be easier to move them as follows:

- Unbutton the coat or jacket.
- Pull the jacket up under the head.
- grasp the jacket under the casualty's shoulders and gently drag them clear.

Carry Chairs

These chairs are used in many shops, schools, hotels and other places of work. They are designed to allow for the evacuation of casualties (or disabled people) up or down stairs and along corridors. Most carry chairs have two or four wheels which makes the movement along flat surfaces much easier. They also have carrying handles for use when going up or down stairs.

Where carry chairs are provided, appropriate training must be given in their use.

- Unfold the chair and test its safety by pressing down on the seat.
- Sit the casualty in the chair and secure the safety harness over the casualty's arms.
- Place the casualty's feet on the foot bar.
- Always support the back of the chair to prevent it from tipping backward.

Moving (one first aider)

- Reassure the casualty and explain what you are going to do.
- If the chair has four wheels, simply push it forward at a controlled speed.
- If the chair has only two rear wheels, carefully tip the chair back and push it forward at a controlled speed, continually reassuring the casualty.

X Do not pull the chair.

Down stairs (only with help)

A casualty who is being moved up or down stairs in a carry chair will feel very insecure and anxious; therefore, reassure them throughout the procedure.

- Stand behind the chair, facing down the stairs. The helper should stand a few steps down, facing the chair.
- Gently tip the chair back and the helper should now firmly grasp the carrying handles on the foot bar.
- On the command of the helper, the chair is lifted.
- The helper should control the pace of the journey down the stairs, step by step.

Up Stairs

- Reverse the procedure.

Test Your Knowledge

1) Give three principles of safe moving:

   i ....

   ii ....

   iii ....

After an An Accident at Work

In addition to providing treatments, the first aider is also responsible for dealing with the 'aftermath' of an accident at work.

There are three tasks which must be performed immediately after an accident at work:

1. Tidying up.
2. Recording details of the accident and any treatments given.
3. Re-stocking the first aid box (this is covered in section 23).

Tidying Up

(As HIV and Hepatitis B Virus stay active for considerable periods of time in dried blood, it is important for employees to be aware of their company's code of practice for dealing with spillages, etc.)

There are two types of waste material which may be produced when dealing with a casualty at work, routine waste and clinical waste.

Routine Waste

This relates to any paper or wrapping from first aid equipment which has been used. If it is uncontaminated, it should simply be put into the normal waste bin.

Clinical Waste

This relates to any items contaminated by the casualty's blood, vomit, saliva or urine. It is improper and potentially unsafe to put this type of waste into the normal bin as it may contain a considerable risk of biological hazard. Clinical waste requires specific management.

- Wear disposable gloves, and apron to protect your clothing.
- If there is spillage of blood, vomit or urine on the floor, it should be disinfected with a suitable solution. There are many proprietary brands of disinfection solution available from medical wholesalers and high street shops. It is often best to use a powdered form of disinfectant rather than a liquid as this will soak up the spillage, not spread it further.

When using disinfectant solution, always follow the advice on the container and, if necessary, wear protective goggles.

- Contaminated dressings, material and paper packets should be carefully placed into a polythene bag. Remember to put your gloves and apron into the bag before sealing it up.
- Yellow bags, as used in first aid-rooms, should be disposed of by incineration.This must be performed in a proper clinical incinerator and not on a makeshift bonfire in the company car park.

  There are two possible ways of ensuring that it is dealt with correctly:

  - If available at work, have the bag put into the sanitary towel waste bin in the ladies toilet. Contract cleaners will now remove the clinical waste from the premises in the correct manner and ensure its safe incineration.
  - Contact your Council or local authority who usually offer a collection service for this type of low-grade, small-quantity biological waste.

Recording Details

It is a legal requirement that details of all accidents in the workplace are recorded in an appropriate manner (this even includes accidents where no one was injured). In many cases, this simply involves filling in the accident book or other suitable in-house form which your company may provide.

The first aider must be able to maintain a simple, factual record of any and all treatments which they have administered at work (even if the only treatment possible was advice to the casualty).

Good record keeping provides a detailed and accurate account of all details relating to the accident and injuries sustained, and this is necessary for many reasons:

- it will allow the employer to evaluate the effectiveness of existing safety policies and procedures;
- it may indicate to the employer the need for new safety policies and procedures (the employer cannot take steps to prevent further accidents and injuries happening if they are unaware of their initial occurrence);

- it may be used as documentary evidence in any legal proceedings concerning compensation, or negligence by the employer or employee.

General Points on Recording and Reporting Accidents

- It is essential that the first aider is familiar with the location of documents used in their own workplace and how to complete them correctly.

- As an absolute minimum, the following details should always be recorded:
  - full name and address of the person who suffered an accident;
  - their occupation;
  - the date when the entry was made;
  - the date and time of the accident;
  - the place and circumstances of the accident, stating clearly the work process which was being performed at the time of the accident;
  - details of any injuries suffered and any treatment given;
  - signature of the person making the entry and their address.
- All details should be written in pen and should be neat and legible.
- Be specific with details relating to the location of injuries, for example '1cm cut to middle finger of left hand' is much more specific than 'cut finger'.
- If ever in doubt about how to record any details, seek the advice of your manager or supervisor.
- If a casualty is so bad that they have to go to their doctor or hospital, inform your manager or supervisor verbally as soon as possible. In some cases, further reporting of the accident to an enforcing authority may be necessary under RIDDOR Regulations (see section 1).

Test Your Knowledge

1) As a "First Aid at Work" designated first aider, you may have to maintain records:

   a) What records are required to be kept by law? ....

   b) Give 2 reasons why it is important to keep records:

      i ....

      ii ....

2) After you have cleaned an area where blood has been spilled, what solution of bleach to water do you use?

   .... part/s bleach to .... part/s water

3) Which of the following does not need reporting under RIDDOR (please tick one answer):

   a) Spinal fracture
   b) An injury that involved the employee being off work for four days
   c) A car accident on the way to work resulting in the death of an employee
   d) A doctor reports to the employer that an employee has a work-related disease of a contagious nature

First-Aid Equipment

Maintaining a suitable and adequate supply of first-aid equipment, based on the needs of the particular workplace, is essential.

Information in this section is taken from the Health and Safety (First-Aid) Regulations 1981 and the accompanying Approved Code of Practice and Guidance

The Health and Safety (First-Aid) Regulations 1981 require every employer to:

"...ensure that there are provided, such equipment and facilities as are adequate and appropriate in the circumstances for enabling first aid to be rendered to his employees if they are injured or become ill at work".

How much first-aid provision an employer has to make depends on the circumstances in each workplace. No fixed level exists, but each employer needs to assess what facilities (and personnel) are appropriate.

When the assessment of first-aid requirements has been completed, the employer should provide the materials, equipment and facilities needed to ensure that the level of cover identified as necessary will be available to employees at all relevant times. This will include ensuring that first-aid equipment, suitably marked and easily accessible, is available in all places where working conditions require it.

First-Aid Containers

The minimum level of first-aid equipment is a suitably stocked and properly identified first-aid container. Every employer should provide for each work site at least one first-aid container, supplied with a sufficient quantity of first-aid materials suitable for the particular circumstances.

First-aid containers should be easily accessible and placed, if possible, near to hand-washing facilities. Employers assessing the need for first-aid provision on large sites should consider providing more than one first-aid container. The container should protect the equipment from dust and damp and should only be stocked with items useful for giving first aid.

Tablets and medications should not be kept, nor should equipment for which the first aider has not been trained in its use.

The container must be identified by a white cross on a green background.

There is no mandatory list of items that should be included in a first-aid container but, as a guide, where no special risk arises in the workplace, a minimum stock of first-aid items would normally be:

- a leaflet giving general guidance on first aid;
- twenty individually wrapped sterile adhesive dressings in assorted sizes. These should be appropriate to the type of work (dressings may be of a detectable type for food handlers);
- two sterile eye pads;
- four individually wrapped triangular bandages (preferably sterile);
- six safety pins;
- six medium-sized individually wrapped sterile unmedicated wound dressings - approximately 12cm x 12cm;
- two large-sized individually wrapped sterile unmedicated wound dressings - approximately 18cm x 18cm;
- one pair of disposable gloves.

This is a suggested contents list only; equivalent but different items will be considered acceptable.

The contents of first-aid containers should be checked at least once a week, and should be re-stocked as soon as possible after use. Sufficient supplies should be held in a back-up stock on site.

Care should be taken to discard items safely after the expiry date has passed.

Additional First-Aid Equipment

The assessment may conclude that there is a need for additional materials and equipment: for example, resuscitation barrier devices, scissors, adhesive tape, disposable aprons and individually wrapped moist wipes. These may be kept in the first-aid container if there is room, but they may be stored separately as long as they are available for use if required.

In particular circumstances, the assessment may identify a need for items such as protective equipment, in case, for example, first aiders have to enter dangerous atmospheres; or blankets to protect casualties from the elements. These additional items should be securely stored near the first-aid container, in the first-aid room or in the hazard area, as appropriate. It is important that access to these items is restricted to people trained in their use.

Where mains tap water is not readily available for eye irrigation, at least a litre of sterile water or sterile normal saline (0.9%) in sealed, disposable containers should be provided. Once the seal has been broken, the contents should not be kept for re-use. The container should not be used after the expiry date.

Travelling First-Aid Kits

First-aid kits for travelling workers would typically contain:

- a leaflet giving general guidance on first aid;
- six individually wrapped sterile adhesive dressings;
- one large sterile unmedicated dressing - approximately 18cm x 18cm;
- two triangular bandages;
- two safety pins;
- individually wrapped moist cleansing wipes;
- one pair of disposable gloves.

This is a suggested contents list only; equivalent but different items will be considered acceptable. As with first-aid containers, the contents of kits should be kept stocked from the back-up stock at the home site.

First-Aid Rooms

Employers should provide a suitable first-aid room or rooms where the assessment of first-aid needs identifies this as necessary. The first-aid room should contain essential first-aid facilities and equipment, be easily accessible to stretchers and be clearly signposted and identified by white lettering or symbols on a green background. If possible, the room should be reserved exclusively for giving first aid.

A first-aid room will usually be necessary in establishments with high risks, such as shipbuilding firms, chemical industries or large construction sites and in larger premises at a distance from medical services. A designated person should be given responsibility for the room.

To be effective, first-aid rooms should:

- be large enough to hold a couch, with enough space at each side for people to work, a desk, a chair and any necessary additional equipment;
- have washable surfaces and adequate heating, ventilation and lighting;
- be kept clean, tidy, accessible and available for use at all times when employees are at work;
- be positioned as near as possible to a point of access for transport to hospital;
- display a notice on the door advising of the names, locations and, if appropriate, telephone extensions of first aiders and how to contact them.

Typical examples of the facilities and equipment a first-aid room may contain are:

- a sink with hot and cold running water;
- drinking water and disposable cups;
- soap and paper towels;
- a store for first-aid materials;
- an adequate supply of first-aid materials, similar in type to those kept in the first-aid container. Remember, a first aider should only use equipment in which they have been trained;
- foot-operated refuse containers, lined with yellow clinical waste bags or a container suitable for the safe disposal of clinical waste;
- a couch with waterproof protection and clean pillows and blankets;
- a chair;
- a telephone or other communication equipment;
- a record book for recording incidents where first aid has been given.

If the first-aid room cannot be reserved exclusively for giving first aid, employers need to take care that the first-aid facilities can be made available quickly if necessary. For example, they should consider the implications of whether:

- the activities usually carried out in the room can be stopped immediately in an emergency;
- the furnishings and equipment can be moved easily and quickly to a position that will not interfere with giving first aid;
- the storage arrangements for first-aid furnishings and equipment allow them to be made quickly available when necessary.

The contents of the first-aid room should be checked on a regular basis, e.g. once a week and re-stocked as soon as possible. Date-expired items should be carefully discarded.

Re-supply of First-Aid Equipment

It is important that first aiders familiarise themselves with the already-established procedure for the re-supply of first-aid equipment in their workplace.

If there is no such procedure in place, liaise with the employer and formulate one.

There are many possible sources for the purchase and re-supply of first-aid materials and equipment. The approved training organisation who ran your first aid course may sell first-aid equipment as a part of their service, or at least they may be able to recommend a potential source of purchase. Alternatively, look in your local business telephone directory under 'First-Aid Equipment Suppliers'.

Test Your Knowledge

1) Delete from the following the items which should not be found in a first aid box which conforms to Health & Safety guidelines:

a) scissors	b) safety pins	c) antiseptic cream	d) eye pads
e) eye bath	f) medium dressings	g) adhesive dressings	h) extra large dressings
i) tweezers	j) sterile triangulars	k) guidance leaflet	l) large dressings

First Aid and Teamwork

There is a saying "a problem shared is a problem halved" and this is very true for all aspects of medical work, especially the practice of first aid.

Many places of work are of a considerable size and spread of location, with a wide range of hazards. In these instances, it is quite usual to find that the employer has decided to have quite a number of first aiders to ensure that at all times when employees are at work, adequate and appropriate first-aid cover is maintained. With even as few as two first aiders, it is possible to have a 'team' approach, and with larger numbers it is a distinct advantage.

First-aid trainers often receive feedback on Refresher and Re-qualification courses which, summed up, amounts to;

'The loneliness of the first aider'

- being the sole first aider when an emergency arises;
- making important decisions;
- coping with a crisis in a calm manner;
- using skills and knowledge which may not have been practised for months or years;
- dealing with their thoughts and emotions after an emergency at work;
- maybe worrying about what else they could have done.

In other words, just being a normal, conscientious person doing their job, probably extremely well, but without much feedback or support.

How can teamwork best operate?

Putting people doing a similar job together and calling them a team does not automatically work. Getting people together in the first place may be a logistical problem. When meeting, some people often don't gell effectively and struggle for control, thus preventing any positive outcomes from the exercise. People trained by different organisations may have learned the same principles but different philosophies. Giving people an hour, once a month, to meet and talk about first aid in their place of work may only achieve a general chat which people working on different shifts may feel is simply not worth the effort.

Someone (usually the training/personnel/health and safety manager) will have the overall responsibility for first aiders and could manage the following stages of development of their first aid team.

Stage 1 - Choosing the team

- Do this with considerable care. The Health and Safety Executive issue guidance which states that an employer should consider the following factors before appointing a first aider:
  - reliability, disposition and communication skills;
  - aptitude and ability to absorb new knowledge and learn new skills;
  - ability to cope with stressful and physically demanding emergency procedures;
  - normal duties. These should be such that they may be left, to go immediately and rapidly to an emergency.
- Having a short interview procedure after inviting applicants to apply is the best method of selection and can improve the status of first aid generally throughout the company.

Stage 2 - Training the team

- Choose a reputable training organisation and, if possible, ask the trainer to visit your premises to experience your workplace activities. This will help the trainer 'tailor' the training to the exact needs of the employer.
- Send the first aiders in groups to be trained (even if re-qualification is not due at the same time. The benefits of working together on a course are very noticeable.)
- Acknowledge the achievements of the recently successful trainees by displaying the certificates or by putting a congratulatory message on the company notice board or in a newsletter.

Stage 3 - Planning the team development

- Choose a structure to suit your workplace, e.g. two teams, one for the night shift and one for the day shift, or one team which meets monthly at a time when everyone can manage.
- Tell the first aiders what you have in mind and build on their comments and suggestions.

- Decide on a format which will meet the needs of the team, e.g. if the workplace is high risk, they may need plenty of practice of skills relating to specific hazards. In some cases, practising specific scenarios and responses could be beneficial.
- Go in gently. People who have not previously practised or trained together often fear making mistakes in front of others, so introduce informal practice as a choice at first.

Stage 4 - Choosing the venue

- Somewhere quiet and preferably private.
- Somewhere with sufficient floor space for practising skills.
- If possible, a room with access to audio and visual aids such as a television and video (there are many first-aid training videos available to refresh knowledge).

Stage 5 - Developing the team

- Have clear aims and objectives for each session.
- Choose a topic for discussion beforehand and, if possible, produce a written programme so that everyone comes prepared.
- Keep the format informal and the atmosphere relaxed; don't conduct it as a chair-person would.
- Discuss incidents which have recently happened and the actions which were taken.
- Allow time for listening to each other.
- Ask advice of each other in instances where you feel unsure.
- Give praise to each other where necessary.

X Do not:

- laugh unkindly at mistakes;
- criticise;
- dominate the conversation;
- talk about people who are not there;
- forget to go to the meeting.

The benefits of having a good team

It has been mentioned that first aid can seem a lonely and responsibility-laden job for lay people who put themselves forward in good faith for training. For this reason, the benefits have been listed to reflect those of the individual and those of the company.

- For the first aider:
  - skills are kept up to date;
  - confidence is maintained;
  - support is received;
  - first aiders can respond together and share problems;
  - more likely to seek advice and opinion from other first aiders;
  - the quality of their response to an emergency is maintained or even improved.
- For the company:
  - awareness of health and safety in the workplace is promoted;
  - morale of the first aiders is improved and may have a knock-on effect on their work;
  - incidents and accidents are dealt with more effectively.

Your chosen approved training provider will be happy to advise on any aspect of first-aid team building within your company.

For Your Notes

Asthma

Asthma is a condition which causes the airways in the lungs to become inflamed and narrow, making it difficult to breathe. In some cases, it may also cause the airways to secrete a thick mucus which further blocks off the airways.

Asthma attacks can be triggered by a variety of stimuli such as allergies, exercise, dust, cold weather, fumes and smoke, and respiratory infections.

Regular sufferers may have been prescribed medication for the condition. There are two main types of medication, those which prevent attacks and those which relieve symptoms. Most asthma medications are administered by inhaling a powder or spray from a 'puffer' or 'inhaler' device.

The medication which is designed to prevent or reduce the frequency and severity of attacks is usually in a brown inhaler. The casualty will take this medication at certain times of the day as prescribed by their doctor. **This medication is a preventer, and therefore of no use during an actual attack.**

The medication which is designed to relieve symptoms is usually in a blue inhaler. The casualty will take this medication when the symptoms of an attack develop. It works by relaxing the constricting airways and allowing them to re-open. This medication is essential during an attack, therefore most people with asthma will always keep their blue inhaler close to hand.

Recognition

- Difficulty in breathing, usually with a prolonged breathing out phase.
- Wheezing.
- The casualty may cough up a thick white mucus.
- Distress and anxiety.
- There may be difficulty in speaking and the casualty may whisper.
- Blueness of the skin (cyanosis) may become evident, especially of the lips.
- The casualty may become exhausted and, in very rare cases, become unconscious and perhaps stop breathing altogether.

Treatment

- Be calm and reassuring and ask any bystanders to leave the area.
- Allow the casualty to adopt a comfortable position which best facilitates breathing. This is often sitting down, leaning forward and resting on a support. Do not lie the casualty down.
- Ensure a good supply of fresh air is available.
- Loosen any tight or restrictive clothing around the neck or waist and encourage the casualty to breathe slowly and deeply.
- Assist the casualty to locate their 'reliever' medication so that they can use it.
- Monitor for any change in the condition.

If the attack eases and the casualty fully recovers, there is no reason why they should not continue with their normal day's activities, although they should be advised to inform their doctor of their attack.

If the casualty should become unconscious, assess ABC and treat accordingly.

Call for an ambulance if:

- this is the first attack;
- the reliever medication has no effect after 3 minutes;
- the casualty is distressed and/or unable to talk;
- the casualty develops any blueness in the skin (cyanosis);
- the casualty becomes unconscious;
- the casualty is becoming exhausted.

Heart Conditions

The heart is without doubt the most hard-working muscle in the human body. At work, at rest, at play and even in our sleep the heart continues to pump blood around the body, beating on average around one hundred thousand times per day.

All this muscular activity requires a good supply of oxygenated blood and this is delivered to the heart muscle by only three coronary arteries. If these arteries become narrowed or blocked, blood supply to the heart muscle will be reduced and the heart will not beat correctly.

There are two main types of heart condition which a first aider may be called on to attend, angina pectoris and heart attack.

Angina Pectoris

This condition arises when the oxygen needs of the heart muscle exceed the amount which can be supplied via the coronary arteries. It is often caused by the formation of a blockage in the coronary arteries which obstructs the passage of oxygenated blood.

Under normal conditions, the heart muscle will still receive sufficient oxygenated blood despite the obstruction, but if the workload of the heart muscle is increased, the muscle becomes starved of oxygen and the condition develops. If the workload of the heart muscle is reduced, the condition often subsides. In some cases, the casualty may have been prescribed medication for their condition. This medication is often in the form of small tablets or a spray which, when taken, quickly relaxes and opens up the narrowed coronary blood vessels.

Recognition

- History of physical activity or emotional distress, thus increasing the workload of the heart.
- Pain, usually in the centre of the chest but it may spread to the arms (particularly the left) and the jaw. It is often described as a tight or crushing pain.
- Shortness of breath.
- The skin may become pale and the casualty may begin to sweat.
- Possible nausea.
- Generalised weakness of other body muscles.

Treatment

The main aim of treatment is to ease the strain on the heart and, if necessary, obtain further medical aid.

- Sit the casualty down in a comfortable position and reassure them.
- If necessary, assist the casualty to locate their prescribed medication so that they can take it.
- Keep the casualty calm and, if the attack eases within a few minutes, advise them to consult their doctor.
- If the pain does not subside within a few minutes or it returns, treat as for a suspected heart attack and call for an ambulance.

Suspected Heart Attack

A heart attack usually occurs when the blood supply to part of the heart muscle is suddenly reduced (unlike angina pectoris where the reduction is gradual). It is often caused by a blood clot in one of the coronary arteries (coronary thrombosis).

The severity of the heart attack will largely depend on the amount of muscle starved of oxygen. In some cases it may be severe enough to make the heart stop beating but many people do survive heart attacks, especially if treatment is given quickly and effectively.

Recognition

- The casualty may have some history of heart disease or heart condition.
- A very tight, 'vice-like' pain in the centre of the chest which is persistent and not relieved by rest. The pain may radiate to the neck, arms, back and upper abdomen.
- Difficulty in breathing.
- Rapid, weak and usually irregular pulse.
- Pale, clammy skin and blueness of the lips and extremities may develop.
- Dizziness.
- Nausea.

- The casualty may suddenly become unconscious and stop breathing.

Treatment

The main aim of treatment is to reduce the workload of the heart and summon urgent medical aid.

- Make the casualty as comfortable as possible, ideally in a half-sitting position with the head and shoulders well supported and, if possible, with the knees slightly bent. Keep the casualty at absolute rest and avoid any unnecessary movement.
- Ask the casualty if they have any history of this condition and, if so, do they have any medication. If the casualty has medication for angina, help them to locate it so that they can take it.
- Reassure the casualty. Do not confirm or infer that they are having a heart attack as this may cause further panic and worsen the condition.
- Without panic, call for an ambulance.
- If the company nurse or doctor are present, they may decide to administer one aspirin to the casualty, which should be chewed slowly. This will help thin the blood and perhaps increase blood flow past the obstruction in the coronary artery.
- If the casualty becomes unconscious, place them into the recovery position and monitor ABC.

Test Your Knowledge

1) Give three signs of someone suffering from a heart attack:

   i ....

   ii ....

   iii ....

2) Why is a coronary thrombosis dangerous?

   ....

3) Your colleague says he has had bad indigestion this week and is having a serious attack this morning. What action should you take (please tick one answer):

   a) help him to take his favourite remedy

   b) call an ambulance to have the pain checked out in case it's his heart

   c) make an appointment for him to see his GP

   d) advise him to adjust his diet to suit his digestion problems

Stroke

A stroke is a condition in which the blood supply to part of the brain has suddenly and seriously become impaired.

It is usually caused by a blood clot (thrombosis) or ruptured blood vessel in the brain.

The overall severity of a stroke will greatly depend on the particular area of the brain in which the clot or rupture has occurred, thus some strokes are referred to as mild and some as severe.

Strokes are more common in later life and particularly in those who suffer from high blood pressure, although anyone has the potential of having a sudden stroke, even young, seemingly fit people. Signs and symptoms of a stroke are very similar to those of compression (see Section 17) except that the condition develops spontaneously, without an injury.

It is vital, for best chances of recovery, to get the casualty to hospital quickly.

Recognition

- The casualty may develop a sudden, severe headache.
- Confusion, dizziness and possible delirium, affecting speech, balance and co-ordination.
- Weakness or total loss of power and function of parts of the body, often one-sided. (As the casualty to grip both your hands to checks this.)
- The pulse may become irregular, slow and strong.
- Pupils may become unequal and their reaction to light may reduce.
- A "dropped" appearance to one side of the face.
- Nausea and possible vomiting.
- Possible loss of bladder and bowel control.
- The casualty may become unconscious and stop breathing.

Treatment

- If the casualty is conscious, lay them down with the head and shoulders raised and supported.
- If the casualty is unconscious, place them into the recovery position.
- Loosen any tight or restrictive clothing.
- Keep the casualty still and cover them with a blanket or coat to prevent unnecessary heat loss.
- Ensure that any fluids in the mouth e.g. vomit or saliva, can easily drain away. If necessary, gently turn their head to one side to allow drainage. If the casualty is dribbling from the mouth, use a cloth or sterile dressing to wipe it away.
- Reassure the casualty at all times: a stroke is sudden and frightening.
- Monitor level of response, breathing and circulation at regular intervals.
- Call for an ambulance as a priority (even for minor strokes) – do not waste time.

Test Your Knowledge

1) You arrive for a meeting with a colleague to find him collapsed, unable to talk properly, with one side of his face dropped and having been sick. What is your priority (please tick one answer):

a) to call an ambulance
b) to make him comfortable
c) to call for help
d) to put him in the recovery position

2) The signs and symptoms of a stroke are similar to:

a) concussion
b) compression
c) fainting
d) epilepsy

Diabetes

Diabetes is a disorder in which the body is unable to regulate the amount of sugar (glucose) in the blood. This happens when there is a lack of a substance called insulin, which is produced naturally in the pancreas. The function of insulin is to assist in the transportation of blood sugar to the cells where it is used to produce energy.

In general, people who have diabetes are unable to naturally produce a sufficient quantity or quality of insulin to control their blood sugar, but, in the main, they are able to control their condition in other ways, depending on the type of diabetes which has been diagnosed. This may be achieved by:

- attention to a particular diet;
- regulating exercise and strenuous activity;
- certain drugs;
- insulin injections.

Hypoglycaemia

This means low (hypo) sugar (glyc) in the blood (aemia) and is the most common diabetic emergency that a first aider is likely to encounter. It can develop very quickly, even in those whose condition is usually well controlled.

Factors which may lead to a lowering of blood sugar (or a 'hypo') are:

- Taking too much insulin or tablets.
- Insufficient intake of food and drink which contains sugar, e.g. missing a meal.
- Excessive or unexpected exercise.
- Stress.
- Drinking alcohol.
- A high body temperature and fever.

Recognition

This varies with individuals, but general recognition points may include:

In a mild case:

- Hunger.
- Sweating and paleness of the skin.
- Trembling/shaking.
- A tingling sensation in the lips, tongue or hands.
- Blurred vision.
- Light-headedness or giddiness.
- Difficulty in concentrating.
- A slow, strong, bounding pulse with rapid shallow breathing.

In a severe case, all of the above, and also:

- Slurred speech.
- Confusion and unusual behaviour which can sometimes become aggressive.
- Possible loss of consciousness.
- Muscular twitching and convulsions.
- Respiratory and cardiac arrest.

Treatment

The main aim of treatment is to restore the level of sugar in the blood to a satisfactory level as soon as possible.

- Keep the casualty still and reassure them.
- If the casualty is conscious, give them sugary food such as chocolate, sweets, biscuits, glucose tablets, lemonade, or plain water with sugar added. It is obviously important that, although conscious, the casualty is able to swallow the food without causing an airway problem and choking.
- If the casualty responds, give them some more sweet food or drink and stay with them until they are fully recovered. Advise them to consult their doctor or diabetic support team.
- If the casualty shows no sign of improvement or the condition worsens, call for an ambulance.
- If the casualty becomes unconscious, do not give them anything by mouth. Place them into the recovery position and monitor airway, breathing and circulation.

Hyperglycaemia

This means high (hyper) sugar in the blood and is a condition of slow onset, usually taking several hours or even days to develop. To prevent sugar building up in the blood, many people with diabetes take insulin injections or tablets at certain times of the day or night as a matter of routine.

Possible causes of hyperglycaemia are:

- Not taking sufficient insulin injections or tablets.
- Infections.
- Too much sugary food.
- Too little exercise.

Recognition

It is very rare for a first aider to come across a hyperglycaemic emergency because the person usually has plenty of warning and therefore time to take their medication to correct the problem. Recognition points may include:

- Thirst.
- Blurred vision.
- Tiredness, lethargy and drowsiness.
- Stomach pains and nausea.
- Flushed, dry skin.
- Rapid pulse and slow, deep breathing.
- A faint smell of acetone (or nail varnish remover) on the breath.
- Unconsciousness and diabetic coma could follow.

Treatment

- Put the casualty into the recovery position and monitor airway, breathing and circulation.
- Call for an ambulance as soon as possible.

Test Your Knowledge

1) A colleague at work, who is normally good natured and friendly, is acting in an angry and argumentative manner. He seems confused and is pale and sweating. To your knowledge he has not been involved in any accident or upsetting incident.

   a) What do you suspect could be the problem? ....

   b) What action will you take? ....

2) People with diabetes sometimes suffer from hypoglycaemia. Give two causes of this condition:

   i ....

   ii ....

Epilepsy & Convulsions

Seizures and convulsions are caused by an abnormal chemical state in the brain and result in bursts of unwanted electrical activity going to other parts of the brain and other parts of the body.

The most common causes of seizures include:

- Epilepsy.
- Poisoning.
- Head Injury.
- An abnormally high rise in body temperature.

Epileptic Seizures

Epilepsy is a disorder or condition, not a disease or mental illness. People who have epilepsy show a tendency to have recurrent seizures (fits).

There are many different ways that epilepsy can be caused, which include brain damage at birth, head injury, stroke and tumours, although for over 50 per cent of people diagnosed with epilepsy, the cause cannot be identified.

Epileptic seizures may be stimulated by certain factors or 'triggers'. Common triggers of epileptic seizures include:

- Lack of food.
- Lack of sleep.
- Alcohol.
- Stress.
- Missed meals.
- Flashing/flickering light.

Types of Epileptic Seizure

Until a few years ago, seizures were classified into two basic groups referred to as 'petit mal' and 'grand mal' meaning small or large seizures. Today, however, much more is known about epilepsy and there is now an international classification system, based on seizure type.

Partial Epileptic Seizures

As the name suggests, partial seizures occur in a localised area of the brain. The nature of the seizure will depend on the particular area of the brain which is affected. There are two main types of partial seizure, simple and complex.

During simple partial seizures awareness is maintained and the person may experience symptoms such as numbness, tingling, sensations of fear, a feeling of nausea, a strange smell or taste. These symptoms are often referred to as an 'aura'.

During complex partial seizures, the person will not be fully alert or aware of their surroundings. The person may demonstrate strange behaviour or symptoms such as lip-smacking, chewing, rubbing of the hands, fiddling with clothing and objects, repetitive speech, mumbling, walking around as if in a trance and they may fall over and incontinence may occur.

Generalised Epileptic Seizures

These involve a disturbance of chemical and electrical activity throughout the whole brain. They can develop on from a partial seizure.

Absences (petit mal) are brief periods of unconsciousness, sometimes with a blank, staring look, fluttering of the eyelids and head nodding. They may only last a few seconds.

Tonic seizures result in a stiffening of the muscles but without jerking. The person may fall to the ground and injury may occur.

Atonic seizures cause a loss of muscle tone and the person becomes floppy. If they are standing, this will result in a heavy fall to the ground. They are often referred to as 'drop attacks'.

Tonic clonic (tightening and jerking) is perhaps the most dramatic form of seizure and is the type which most people relate to epilepsy. The person initially becomes rigid and, if standing, will fall to the ground. Jerking of the limbs will follow, usually with noisy or interrupted breathing. This may cause cyanosis (blueness of the lips and skin due to lack of oxygen). Saliva and nasal mucus may froth around the nose and mouth, which could be bloodstained if the tongue or cheek has been bitten during the seizure. In some cases, the person may become incontinent. The seizure may last from just a few seconds to a few minutes. Afterwards, the person will feel very tired and may go into a deep sleep.

Non-Epileptic Seizures and Convulsions

Seizures and convulsions may be caused by other factors apart from epilepsy, although they may show similar recognition points. Common causes of non-epileptic seizures include head injuries, poisoning and an abnormally high rise in body temperature.

Management of Seizures and Convulsions

During a seizure (regardless of type or cause), the main aim of treatment is to ensure that the person does not injure themselves.

- If consciousness has not been lost, talk to the person in a calm and reassuring way and, if necessary, try to guide them away from any danger. Do not try to restrain their movements. When fully recovered, reassure the person and give assistance where necessary.
- If consciousness has been fully lost, protect the person from harm. If necessary, move any objects from the surrounding area and try to protect the head from banging against the ground. Do not try to restrict any movements and do not put anything in the person's mouth.
- In all cases, try to ensure privacy by asking onlookers to leave the area.
- When the seizure is over, ensure the airway is clear and open, and check for breathing. Assess the person for any injuries and place them into the recovery position. Cover the person with a coat or blanket and stay with them until they have fully recovered.
- Always respect the privacy and dignity of a person who is having, or has had, a seizure.
- In cases where epilepsy is the cause of the seizure, make a note of the duration of the seizure and pass this information to the casualty when they recover.

Calling for an Ambulance

It is not always necessary to call for an ambulance if the person is known to have epilepsy. However, the emergency services should be called if:

- the seizure is not thought to be due to epilepsy (e.g. there is evidence of head injury, poisoning or harmful substances);
- the seizure shows no sign of stopping after a few minutes;
- the seizure stops but is followed by another seizure without any time for recovery between;
- injury has occurred which will require further medical attention;
- if the person is not known to have had seizures before;
- if the person does not show signs of recovery from unconsciousness after 10 minutes.

Test Your Knowledge

1) You are called to deal with someone who is known to have epilepsy and who is now having a 'major' seizure.

    a) What will you do when the convulsions have ceased? ....

    ....

b) Give three circumstances when you should call an ambulance to attend a casualty suffering from epilepsy.

    i ....

    ii ....

    iii ....

Allergic Reactions

Allergic reaction is a condition where the body reacts to an unwelcome 'foreign' substance (usually protein based). Common substances which may cause an allergic reaction include:

- Bites and stings, from insects, snakes, jellyfish and plants.
- Drugs, such as penicillin.
- Pollen.
- Animal dust and hairs.
- Certain materials such as latex.
- Certain foodstuffs such as nuts, eggs and shellfish.

Most people have a normal defence mechanism to protect them from foreign substances and micro-organisms that do not belong in the body. The main defence is the release of chemicals to neutralise the foreign substance. The most prominent chemical released is called histamine. The presence of histamine, and many other chemicals, very quickly renders the foreign substance harmless and the person continues their activities none the wiser and no worse for the experience.

The problem with allergies is not, as one may suspect, due to the non-release of a chemical and histamine response, but quite the opposite. In some people the chemical and histamine release in response to the invading foreign substance is much higher than required and the over-release of histamine itself becomes a problem, causing localised and generalised effects which in extreme cases can become life-threatening.

People who suffer from allergic reactions are often prescribed anti-histamine drugs by their doctor. These drugs reduce the person's release of histamine to an acceptable level.

Mild Allergic Reaction

This is when only a small over-release of histamine occurs.

Recognition

- The casualty may know that they have an allergy. If they don't tell you, ask.
- A localised skin reaction may develop such as a rash, blotches and slight swelling. This is often very itchy.
- The eyes may puff up and begin to water.
- Membranes at the back of the nose and throat may become irritable, causing a runny nose and sneezing.
- Other mild symptoms may be present which are specific to the particular casualty.

Treatment

- If possible, try to move the casualty away from the substance causing the allergic reaction.
- Ask the casualty if they need to take any prescribed medication for the allergy.
- Reassure the casualty at all times.
- Apply a cold compress to areas of the skin which are red, swollen or itchy.
- If the reaction does not subside within 30 minutes or the reaction worsens, call for further medical assistance.
- Advise the casualty to see their doctor.

Severe Allergic Reaction

Although rare, some people do have an overwhelming release of histamine in response to foreign substances. This is called anaphylactic shock. In large amounts, this histamine overdose causes two main problems.

1. It causes the bronchi and bronchioles in the lungs to constrict, thus narrowing the airways and making breathing very difficult.
2. The heart muscle is weakened and the output of blood from the heart is reduced. This causes a marked reduction in blood pressure.

If a person is known to suffer from anaphylactic shock, their doctor may have prescribed a drug called adrenalin (epinephrin) which they carry on their person for their use during an attack. This medication comes in the form of an automatic injection device (often called an epi-pen). Adrenalin injection has many beneficial effects for a casualty in anaphylactic shock although it is stressed that the first aider should not attempt to administer the drug unless they are authorised and trained to do so.

Recognition

- The casualty may tell you of a history of allergy. If they don't tell you, ask.

- A localised or generalised skin reaction may develop such as a rash, blotches and severe swelling.
- The eyes, lips and tongue may begin to swell.
- The casualty may develop a tightness in the chest, making breathing very difficult (this often resembles a severe asthma attack).
- The casualty may become dizzy and light-headed due to a lack of blood and oxygen to the brain.
- Abdominal cramps and vomiting may be present and, in later stages, diarrhoea may develop.
- The casualty may lose consciousness.
- Respiratory and cardiac arrest may follow.

Treatment.

- Carry out the ABC of emergency diagnosis.

If the casualty is conscious:

- Help the casualty into a position which most relieves any breathing difficulty and loosen any tight or restrictive clothing.
- Reassure the casualty at all times.
- If the casualty carries an epi-pen, you may assist them to locate it, but remember, you must not perform the injection yourself unless you are authorised and trained to do so.
- Use a cold compress to reduce any swelling around the neck or throat.
- Call for an ambulance as soon as possible and pass on any details regarding the casualty's condition.

If the casualty becomes unconscious:

- Place them into the recovery position and monitor breathing and pulse.
- Call for an ambulance.
- If circulation or breathing should stop, carry out resuscitation.

For Your Notes

Hyperventilation

Hyperventilation (or over-breathing) may often result from a panic attack where the casualty is subject to a high degree of emotional distress.

In many cases, the casualty may be unaware that they are hyperventilating and a firm but friendly manner is required during treatment.

Hyperventilation results in too much carbon dioxide being lost from the body and a rise in the amount of oxygen in the blood stream. The fall in carbon dioxide levels in the blood stream causes blood vessels in the brain to constrict. This, in turn, further reduces the oxygen supply to the brain tissues and may eventually result in unconsciousness.

Recognition

- A history of emotional distress, anxiety or panic.
- The breathing rate and depth will change. It usually starts fast and shallow, gradually becoming stronger and deeper.
- There may be muscular spasms and stiffening of hands and feet.
- The casualty may feel light-headed, dizzy and may have a tingling 'pins and needles' sensation or numbness over the body.
- Possible unconsciousness.

Treatment

The main aim of treatment is to correct the levels of oxygen and carbon dioxide in the casualty's blood.

- Move the casualty to a private and quiet area if possible.
- Reassure and speak to the casualty in a firm and reassuring manner.
- Advise the casualty to slow down and regulate their breathing with conscious control.
- If tingling or muscular spasms continue, it may help if the casualty breathes into and out of a paper bag. This will increase the amount of inspired carbon dioxide and reduce the amount of inspired oxygen.
- On recovery, continue to reassure the casualty and, if appropriate, advise them to seek further qualified attention for any underlying emotional distress or medical condition.
- If symptoms persist for more than a few minutes or if the casualty becomes unconscious, call for an ambulance.

For Your Notes

First Aid for Children

Some first aiders work in premises where children are present, perhaps in a shop, school, cinema or sports centre. It is therefore essential that these first aiders have a knowledge of the modifications to adult first aid which are necessary when dealing with children and infants.

One of the major considerations when dealing with injured or sick children is their general inability to communicate effectively, particularly when trying to tell you what is wrong and especially when they are crying. This means that the first aider should be patient and understanding throughout treatment and care, and may need to ask the parent or carer if the child is normally as quiet as this, for example.

Choking and Obstructed Airway

For a Child (one to eight years of life)

- If the child is breathing spontaneously, their efforts to clear the obstruction should be encouraged. Intervention is only necessary if these attempts are clearly ineffective and breathing is inadequate.

If intervention is deemed necessary:

- Do not perform blind finger sweeps of the mouth or upper airway – this could either push the object further in or damage the soft tissue inside the child's mouth.
- Sit down and lay the child across your lap, face down with the head lower than their body. Because of gravity, this position will help the object fall from the mouth.
- Give five slaps with the flat of the hand to the middle of the back, between the shoulder blades.

If the object is not dislodged, proceed to chest thrusts.

- Stand or kneel behind the child and put your arms around his chest.
- Give five chest thrusts on the breastbone in the same position as for chest compressions. Chest thrusts are similar to chest compressions but they should be sharper and more vigorous, at a rate of one every three seconds.
- After five back blows and five chest thrusts, check the mouth and remove any visible obstruction.
- If chest thrusts fail, put your arms around his upper abdomen. Grasping your fist, try up to five abdominal thrusts between the navel and the bottom of the breastbone.
- If obstruction still has not cleared, start whole sequence again with five slaps to the back. Ensure ambulance is called.
- Continue until help arrives or child becomes unconscious.
- If child becomes unconscious give 2 rescue breaths – try up to 5 attempts. If not effective, immediately start chest compressions and continue using CPR sequence described below.

For an Infant (under one year of age)

The procedure is the same as the sequence above but without the use of abdominal thrusts. (Abdominal thrusts are not recommended for infants due to the extensive internal damage they may cause).

- Carry out cycles of five back blows and five chest thrusts only, until the infant breathes spontaneously or the airway is cleared. (Chest thrusts should be carried out on a flat surface.)

Resuscitation

For the purposes of resuscitation, an infant is aged under one year old and a child is between one and eight years of age. Children over the age of eight will still be treated as for a younger child but may require different techniques to attain adequate chest compressions.

In general, the resuscitation procedures for children and infants are similar to those of adults (see section 8) but some modifications are required.

- Check for danger and shout for help.
- Open the airway using the head tilt - chin lift (but be very gentle to avoid injury to the neck).
- Check for breathing (up to 10 seconds).
- If signs of breathing are absent, remove any obvious obstruction from the mouth, take a breath and give up to five rescue breaths, each of which makes the chest rise and fall. A minimum of two effective breaths should be given.

  If the casualty is a child, pinch the nostrils and use mouth to mouth ventilation. If the casualty is an infant, use mouth to mouth and nose (it is very awkward pinching an infant's nostrils so place your mouth over the infant's mouth and nose). Note any gag or cough response to your action.

If rescue breathing is unsuccessful, re-position the airway and try again. If still unsuccessful, the airway may be obstructed (refer to airway obstruction in this section).

- Assess for circulation. Take no more than 10 seconds to:
  - Look for any movement, coughing or normal breathing (more than the occasional gasp).
  - Check for a pulse (if you are a health care provider):

    In a child - by feeling for the carotid pulse in the neck.

    In an infant - by feeling for the brachial pulse in the inner aspect of the upper arm.
- If you are confident that you can detect signs of circulation within ten seconds, continue rescue breathing, if necessary, until they begin to breathe for themselves, then turn into the recovery position if they remain unconscious.
- If there are no signs of circulation, or you are at all unsure, (or in infants if the pulse rate is very slow, i.e. less than one beat per second), combine rescue breathing with chest compressions.

For a child (below 8 years of age):

- Locate and place the heel of one hand over the lower half of the sternum, ensuring that you do not compress on the very bottom of the sternum or below.
- Lift the fingers to ensure that pressure is not applied over the ribs.
- Position yourself vertically above the child's chest, and with your arms straight, press down on the sternum to depress it approximately one third the depth of the child's chest.
- Release the pressure, then repeat at a rate of about 100 per minute (a little less than two compressions per second).
- After five compressions, open the airway and give one effective breath of mouth to mouth ventilation.
- Continue chest compressions and breaths in a ratio of 5 to 1.

For a child (above 8 years of age):

It may be necessary to use the 'adult', two handed method.

- Locate the lower half of the sternum and place the heel of one hand there, with the other hand placed on top.
- Interlock the fingers of both hands and lift them to ensure that pressure is not applied over the child's ribs.
- Position yourself vertically above the child's chest, and with your arms straight, press down on the sternum to depress it approximately one third the depth of the child's chest.
- Release the pressure, then repeat at a rate of about 100 per minute (a little less than two compressions per second).
- After fifteen compressions, open the airway and give two effective breaths of mouth to mouth ventilation.
- Continue chest compressions and breaths at a ratio of 15 to 2.

For an infant:

- Locate the sternum and place the tips of two fingers, one finger breadth below an imaginary line joining the infant's nipples.
- With the tips of two fingers, press down on the sternum to depress it approximately one third the depth of the infant's chest.
- Release the pressure, then repeat at a rate of about 100 per minute (a little less than two compressions per second).
- After five compressions, open the airway and give one effective breath of mouth to mouth and nose ventilation.
- Continue chest compressions and breaths in a ratio of 5 to 1.
- In all cases, continue resuscitation until:

  The child shows signs of life (spontaneous respiration and pulse).

  Qualified help arrives.

  You become exhausted.
- It is vital for rescuers to get help as quickly as possible when a child collapses, so:
  - If more than one rescuer is available, one should start resuscitation while the other rescuer goes for help.
  - If only one rescuer is available, they should perform resuscitation for approximately one minute before going for assistance. It may be possible to take an infant or small child with you whilst summoning help.

Recovery Position

With children, it is often easy to place them into the recovery position (rather than pull them into it) because of their smaller size.

With infants, cradle the infant in your arms with the head tilting downwards to prevent the tongue or vomit from obstructing the airway. If you lay the infant down on their side, you will need to position a rolled up blanket or small pillow behind their back to keep them stable.

Convulsions

A convulsion is a fit or seizure (see appendix E). In infants and children the cause of convulsions may be due to:

- A sudden rise in temperature because they have an infection which causes fever such as influenza.
- An infection of the brain or spinal cord tissues, such as encephalitis or meningitis.
- They are too hot (e.g. in their winter clothes in a warm department store, an overheated car or on a sunny day).
- Epilepsy.
- Poisoning.

Treatment

- Follow the treatment for epilepsy until the convulsion is finished and do not leave the child on their own.
- When the convulsion is over and the child is sleepy, make sure they are on their side in the recovery position.
- If the convulsions were due to a high temperature, take off their clothing to allow cooling. To lower the temperature further, it may be necessary to sponge them down with tepid (not cold) water. Dry them thoroughly and replace some of the clothing.
- In all cases of children having unusual convulsions, call for a doctor or dial 999 for further help.

Shock

Children experience shock every time an accident happens. They may cry loudly, want their mummy or daddy and they may cling to their carer. They need cuddles and lots of reassurance, sometimes for even the most minor mishap.

In some cases, they may go pale and weak for a short period of time but usually get better quickly after a cuddle from mummy or daddy. First aiders, however, should respect good practice, and children should only be cuddled by their parents or carer.

It often helps during the reassurance to try to take the child's mind off the problem, perhaps by telling them a story or giving them a favourite soft toy to cuddle.

If a child has serious shock which is due to a physical injury rather than emotional distress, they should be treated as for adults (see section 11) and an ambulance should be called for urgently. Never leave an injured child alone.

Important points to remember with children:

- Do not shake children to get a response – tap the shoulder
- Children suffer mild shock much more easily than adults
- Never leave a child who is injured alone
- First aiders should respect good professional practice - don't cuddle children who are not yours - let the parents do this
- It can be harrowing dealing with a screaming child: try to distance yourself from this, reassure the child and keep calm to ensure you work quickly in the child's interests
- Anticipate shock if there is blood loss or a burn or scald and treat the child as well as the injury
- Some children fall and injure internal organs or bones without immediate, obvious effect
- Treat an unusually quiet child who has had an accident with no obvious signs of an injury as a shocked child and get them to hospital quickly

For Your Notes

Index

THE FIRST AIDER IN THE WORKPLACE

A Suggested Job Description

To take charge at the scene of an accident at work in the absence of any other suitably qualified person. This may include:

- ✓ assessing for, and dealing with, any hazards/dangers which may be present at the scene
- ✓ delegating responsibilities to others at the scene

To respond to the needs of injured or sick people in the workplace. This may include:

- ✓ assessing an injured or sick person and determining (to the best of their ability) the injury/condition from which they are suffering
- ✓ if possible, providing simple treatment to an injured/sick person within the confines of basic first-aid practice
- ✓ giving basic and appropriate advice to an injured/sick person in relation to the injury/condition from which they are suffering
- ✓ if appropriate to the case, ensuring that injured or sick people are transferred to further medical help of a professional capacity and within a time-frame appropriate to the circumstances

To deal with the "aftermath" having responded to an accident or incident in the workplace. This may include:

- ✓ tidying up and clearing away after an accident
- ✓ monitoring the hygienic disposal of spillages and waste material
- ✓ always writing up simple but complete factual records of accidents and treatments given

In liaison with the employer, to ensure that an adequate stock of appropriate first-aid equipment and materials is maintained in the workplace.

(A sick person could be someone who has a medical condition which comes on suddenly and could have potentially life-threatening consequences – or someone who has a minor illness of a localised nature.)